Clinical Pharmacokinetics

Clinical Pharmacokinetics

Edited by

Soraya Dhillon

BPharm, PhD, MRPharmS

Head of School,
The School of Pharmacy, University of Hertfordshire,
Hatfield, UK

Andrzej Kostrzewski

BSc, MSc, MMedEd, MRPharmS, ILTM

Senior Principal Pharmacist/Academic Manager in Clinical Pharmacy
Education & Development Unit, Pharmacy Department
Guy's Hospital,
London
and The School of Pharmacy, University of Hertfordshire,
Hatfield, UK

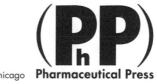

London • Chicago **Pharmaceutical Press**

Published by the Pharmaceutical Press
An imprint of RPS Publishing

1 Lambeth High Street, London SE1 7JN, UK
100 South Atkinson Road, Suite 206, Grayslake, IL 60030-7820, USA

© Pharmaceutical Press 2006

(**PP**) is a trade mark of RPS Publishing

RPS Publishing is the wholly-owned publishing organisation of the Royal
Pharmaceutical Society of Great Britain

Typeset by Gray Publishing, Tunbridge Wells, Kent
Printed in Great Britain by TJ International, Padstow, Cornwall

ISBN-10 0 85369 571 7
ISBN-13 978 0 85369 571 4

A catalogue record for this book is available from the British Library

Contents

Preface

Effective use of medicines requires the pharmacist to have a clear understanding of the principles of drug handling. This knowledge basis is vital to ensure that patients receive the most appropriate drug regimen. The pharmacist's unique knowledge base of drug formulation, pharmacokinetics and factors influencing drug handling is required to ensure the appropriate use of medicines in clinical practice. In clinical practice most drugs that require the application of pharmacokinetics are drugs that show a narrow therapeutic range.

Therapeutic drug monitoring (TDM) is a process of individualising drug therapy through the use of serum drug concentrations and pharmacokinetic and pharmacodynamic concepts. The practical use of TDM skills is fundamental to effective management of patients' medicines. This textbook is designed to be a practical guide to the use of pharmacokinetic principles in clinical practice. The authors come from a range of backgrounds and the contribution of their experiences from many years of formal postgraduate education in pharmacokinetics and bedside medicine management has motivated the character of this book. The book is intended to be used as a practical tool to aid the solving of pharmacokinetic problems in real life and as an aid for undergraduate studies. This subject should not be learnt in isolation from therapeutics at the bedside. There are very few practical pharmacokinetic texts available that do not use complicated multicompartmental mathematical equations; this is one of them. It is not intended to create a fully competent practitioner in clinical pharmacokinetics, but it will provide an important and practical orientation to the concepts involved and how they can be used in the clinical setting.

The aim of the book is to facilitate the use of basic pharmacokinetic concepts close to the patient in daily practice. It is directed at postgraduates in the workplace, to be used as a resource for addressing the gap between theory and art of practice. It will also be a useful tool for undergraduates and clinical tutors.

Soraya Dhillon
Andrzej Kostrzewski
February 2006

About the editors

Soraya Dhillon
Professor Soraya Dhillon is Head of the recently established School of
Pharmacy at the University of Hertfordshire, Hatfield, UK. She is a quali-
fied pharmacist and holds a PhD in pharmacology. Her PhD and research
interests are in the field of pharmacokinetics. Professor Dhillon was responsible for establishing one of the first pharmacokinetic therapeutic drug
level monitoring services in the UK at Northwick Park Hospital, Harrow,
London. She has over 20 years' experience of teaching pharmacokinetics
at undergraduate and postgraduate level and has also published extensively in clinical pharmacokinetics.

Andrzej Kostrzewski
Andrzej Kostrzewski is a Senior Clinical Pharmacist working at Guy's and
St Thomas' Hospital, London. He is also the academic lead for Clinical
Pharmacy at the School of Pharmacy, University of Hertfordshire. He has
extensive experience of education and training of pharmacokinetics at
postgraduate level, and is an experienced clinical practitioner with over
20 years' experience in hospital practice.

Both authors were founder members of the Clinical Pharmacokinetics
Society and have run numerous workshops in the UK and overseas on
clinical pharmacokinetics and therapeutic drug level monitoring.

Contributors

Caroline Ashley MSc, BPharm, MRPharmS
Principal Pharmacist, Renal Services, Royal Free Hampstead NHS Trust,
London, UK

Chris Cairns BSc, MSc, FRPharmS
Professor of Pharmacy Practice, Kingston University, School of Pharmacy,
Surrey, UK

Neil A Caldwell BSc, MSc, MRPharmS
Deputy Chief Pharmacist, Clinical Services, Wirral Hospital NHS Trust,
Merseyside and Honorary Lecturer, School of Pharmacy and Chemistry,
Liverpool John Moores University, Liverpool, UK

Judith Cope BPharm, MSc, MRPharmS, CertHealthEcon
Chief Pharmacist, Pharmacy Department, Hospital for Children,
Great Ormond Street, London, UK

Soraya Dhillon BPharm, PhD, MRPharmS
Head of School, The School of Pharmacy, University of Hertfordshire,
Hatfield, UK

Otto Roman Frey PhD
Clinical Pharmacist, Drug Information Specialist, Kliniken des Landkreises
Heidenheim, Pharmacy Department, Heidenheim, Germany

Kiren Gill BSc
Medical student, University College London and Royal Free Medical
School, University of London, UK

Andrzej Kostrzewski BSc, MSc, MMedEd, MRPharmS, ILTM
Senior Principal Pharmacist/Academic Manager in Clinical Pharmacy,
Education & Development Unit, Pharmacy Department, Guy's Hospital,
London and The School of Pharmacy, University of Hertfordshire,
Hatfield, UK

Douglas Maclean BSc, MRPharmS, DipClinPharm
Renal Pharmacist, Pharmacy Department, Guy's Hospital, London, UK

Patricia M Morgan BPharm, MSc, MRPharmS, SP
Principal Pharmacist, Department of Pharmacy, Neville Hall Hospital,
Abergavenny, UK

Graham Mould BPharm, MSc, PhD, MRPharmS
Director of Operations, Guildford Clinical Pharmacology Unit Ltd,
Surrey Technology Centre, Guildford, Surrey, UK

Wiltrud Probst PhD
Clinical Pharmacist, Drug Information Specialist, Kliniken des Landkreises
Heidenheim, Pharmacy Department, Heidenheim, Germany

Mark Tomlin BPharm, MSc, MRPharmS
Consultant Pharmacist: Critical Care, Pharmacy Department,
Southampton General Hospital, Southampton, UK

Caron Weeks BPharm, MRPharmS, DipPharmPrac
Directorate Pharmacist for Medicine and Elderly Care, Pharmacy
Department, Southampton General Hospital, Southampton, UK

Ian Chi Kei Wong BSc, MSc, PhD, MRPharmS, ILTM(HE)
DH National Public Health Career Scientist and Professor of Paediatric
Medicines Research, Centre for Paediatric Pharmacy Research, The School
of Pharmacy, Institute of Child Health and Great Ormond Street Hospital
for Children, London, UK

Abbreviations

α_1-GP	alpha acid glycoprotein
ABW	actual body weight
ADME	absorption, distribution, metabolism, excretion
AF	atrial fibrillation
AIDS	acquired immunodeficiency syndrome
ALP	alkaline phosphatase
ALT	alanine aminotransferase
AST	aspartate aminotransferase
ATP	adenosine triphosphate
AUC	area under the concentration–time curve
AV	atrioventricular
CAPD	continuous ambulatory peritoneal dialysis
CAVH	continuous arteriovenous haemofiltration
CAVHD	continuous arteriovenous haemodiafiltration
CCF	congestive cardiac failure
CNS	central nervous system
COPD	chronic obstructive pulmonary disease
CRRT	continuous renal replacement therapy
CSF	cerebrospinal fluid
CVVH	continuous veno-venous haemofiltration
CVVHD	continuous veno-venous haemodiafiltration
DLIS	digoxin-like immunoreactive substance
DMO	dimethadione
DTPA	diethylenetriamine penta-acetic acid
DUP	drug use process
ECG	electrocardiogram/electrocardiography
ESRF	end-stage renal failure
FDA	Food and Drug Administration
FPIA	fluorescence polarisation immunoassay
GABA	γ-aminobutyric acid
GC	gas chromatography
GFR	glomerular filtration rate
GGT	gamma glutamyl transferase

GSK	glycogen synthase kinase
HD	haemodialysis
HDU	high dependency unit
HPLC	high-pressure liquid chromatography
HRT	hormone replacement therapy
IBW	ideal body weight
ICG	indocyanine green
IHD	intermittent haemodialysis
IHD	ischaemic heart disease
IL-2	interleukin-2
IM	intramuscular(ly)
ITU	intensive therapy unit
IV	intravenous(ly)
JVP	jugular venous pulse
LSS	limited sampling strategy
MARCKS	myristoylated alanine-rich C kinase substrate
MEGX	monoethylglycinexylidide
MHD	10,11-dihydro-10-hydroxy-5*H*-dibenzo(*b,f*)azepine-5-carboxamide
MRSA	methicillin-resistant *Staphylococcus aureus*
MW	molecular weight
NSAIDs	nonsteroidal anti-inflammatory drugs
OTC	over the counter
PD	peritoneal dialysis
PE	phenyotin sodium equivalent
PI	phosphinositide
PKC	protein kinase C
PMH	past medical history
PND	paroxysmal nocturnal dyspnoea
RIA	radioimmunoassay
rINN	Recommended International Nonproprietary Name
SHO	senior house officer
SSRI	selective serotonin reuptake inhibitor
TCM	trough level concentration monitoring
TCR	T-cell receptor
TDM	therapeutic drug monitoring
TIA	transient ischaemic attack
TLC	trough level concentration
TMO	trimethadione
UFR	ultrafiltrate
WBC	white blood cells

Prescription terms:

o.d.	daily
b.d.	twice daily
t.d.s.	three times daily
q.d.s.	four times daily
mane	in the morning
nocte	at night
p.r.n.	when required
stat	immediately

Superscripts/subscripts on pharmacokinetic parameters:

0, 1, 2	time 0, 1, 2
cr	creatinine
Dig	digoxin
Gent	gentamicin
Li	lithium
max	maximum
min	minimum
p	plasma
ss	steady state
t	time

Units:

μg	microgram
bpm	beats per minute
Da	dalton
dL	decilitre
Eq	equivalent
ft	foot/feet
g	gram
h	hour
in.	inch
kg	kilogram
L	litre
mg	milligram
min	minute
mL	millilitre
mol	mole
mol	millimole
ng	nanogram

1

Basic pharmacokinetics

Soraya Dhillon and Kiren Gill

Aims and learning outcomes

Pharmacokinetics is a fundamental scientific discipline that underpins applied therapeutics. Patients need to be prescribed appropriate medicines for a clinical condition. The medicine is chosen on the basis of an evidence-based approach to clinical practice and assured to be compatible with any other medicines or alternative therapies the patient may be taking.

The design of a dosage regimen is dependent on a basic under-standing of the drug use process (DUP). When faced with a patient who shows specific clinical signs and symptoms, pharmacists must always ask a fundamental question: 'Is this patient suffering from a drug-related problem?' Once this issue is evaluated and a clinical diagnosis is avail-able, the pharmacist can apply the DUP to ensure that the patient is prescribed an appropriate medication regimen, that the patient under-stands the therapy prescribed, and that an agreed concordance plan is achieved.

Pharmacists using the DUP consider:

- Need for a drug
- Choice of a drug
- Goals of therapy
- Design of regimen
  - Route
  - Dose and frequency
  - Duration
- Monitoring and review
- Counselling

Once a particular medicine is chosen, the principles of clinical pharmaco-kinetics are required to ensure the appropriate formulation of drug is chosen for an appropriate route of administration. On the basis of the patient's drug handling parameters, which require an understanding of absorption, distribution, metabolism and excretion, the dosage regimen for the medicine in a particular patient can be developed. The pharmacist will then need to ensure that the appropriate regimen is prescribed to achieve optimal efficacy and minimal toxicity. Pharmacists then ensure that the appropriate monitoring is undertaken and that the patient receives the appropriate information to ensure compliance. Clinical pharmacokinetics is thus a fundamental knowledge base that pharmacists require to ensure effective practice of pharmaceutical care.

The aim of this chapter is to provide the practising clinical pharmacist with the appropriate knowledge and skills of applied clinical pharmacokinetics, which can be applied in everyday practice.

The objectives for this chapter are to enable the reader to:

- State the rationale for using therapeutic drug monitoring (TDM) to optimise drug therapy.
- Identify drugs that should be routinely monitored.
- Define first-order and zero-order kinetics.
- Apply one-compartment pharmacokinetics to single and multiple dosing following the intravenous and oral administration of drugs.
- Apply the basic principles of interpretation of serum drug concentrations in practice.
- Apply one-compartment pharmacokinetics to describe steady-state serum drug concentrations following oral slow-release dosing.
- Use the method of iteration to derive individualised pharmacokinetic parameters from serum drug concentration data.
- Apply nonlinear pharmacokinetics to describe steady-state plasma concentrations following parenteral and/or oral phenytoin therapy.

Introduction

Pharmacokinetics provides a mathematical basis to assess the time course of drugs and their effects in the body. It enables the following processes to be quantified:

Absorption
Distribution
Metabolism
Excretion

These pharmacokinetic processes, often referred to as ADME, determine the drug concentration in the body when medicines are prescribed. A fundamental understanding of these parameters is required to design an

Table 1.1 Drugs that should be routinely monitored

Therapeutic group	Drugs
Aminoglycosides	Gentamicin, tobramycin, amikacin
Cardioactive	Digoxin, lidocaine
Respiratory	Theophylline
Anticonvulsant	Phenytoin, carbamazepine, phenobarbital
Others	Lithium, ciclosporin

appropriate drug regimen for a patient. The effectiveness of a dosage regimen is determined by the concentration of the drug in the body.

Ideally, the concentration of drug should be measured at the site of action of the drug; that is, at the receptor. However, owing to inaccessibility, drug concentrations are normally measured in whole blood from which serum or plasma is generated. Other body fluids such as saliva, urine and cerebrospinal fluid (CSF) are sometimes used. It is assumed that drug concentrations in these fluids are in equilibrium with the drug concentration at the receptor.

It should be noted that the measured drug concentrations in plasma or serum are often referred to as drug *levels*, which is the term that will be used throughout the text. It refers to total drug concentration, i.e. a combination of bound and free drug that are in equilibrium with each other.

In routine clinical practice, serum drug level monitoring and optimisation of a dosage regimen require the application of clinical pharmacokinetics. A number of drugs show a narrow therapeutic range and for these drugs therapeutic drug level monitoring is required (Chapter 2). Table 1.1 identifies drugs that should be routinely monitored.

A variety of techniques is available for representing the pharmacokinetics of a drug. The most usual is to view the body as consisting of compartments between which drug moves and from which elimination occurs. The transfer of drug between these compartments is represented by rate constants, which are considered below.

Rates of reaction

To consider the processes of ADME the *rates* of these processes have to be considered; they can be characterised by two basic underlying concepts.

The rate of a reaction or process is defined as the velocity at which it proceeds and can be described as either *zero-order* or *first-order*.

Zero-order reaction

Consider the rate of elimination of drug A from the body. If the amount of the drug, A, is decreasing at a constant rate, then the rate of elimination of A can be described as:

$$\frac{dA}{dt} = -k^*$$

where k^* = the zero-order rate constant.

    The reaction proceeds at a constant rate and is independent of the concentration of A present in the body. An example is the elimination of alcohol. Drugs that show this type of elimination will show accumulation of plasma levels of the drug and hence nonlinear pharmacokinetics.

First-order reaction

If the amount of drug A is decreasing at a rate that is proportional to A, the amount of drug A remaining in the body, then the rate of elimination of drug A can be described as:

$$\frac{dA}{dt} = -kA$$

where k = the first-order rate constant.

    The reaction proceeds at a rate that is dependent on the concentration of A present in the body. It is assumed that the processes of ADME follow first-order reactions and most drugs are eliminated in this manner.

    Most drugs used in clinical practice at therapeutic dosages will show first-order rate processes; that is, the rate of elimination of most drugs will be first-order. However, there are notable exceptions, for example phenytoin and high-dose salicylates. In essence, for drugs that show a first-order elimination process one can show that, as the amount of drug administered increases, the body is able to eliminate the drug accordingly and accumulation will not occur. If you double the dose you will double the plasma concentration. However, if you continue to increase the amount of drug administered then all drugs will change from showing a first-order process to a zero-order process, for example in an overdose situation.

Pharmacokinetic models

Pharmacokinetic models are hypothetical structures that are used to describe the fate of a drug in a biological system following its administration.

One-compartment model

Following drug administration, the body is depicted as a kinetically homogeneous unit (see Figure 1.1). This assumes that the drug achieves instantaneous distribution throughout the body and that the drug equilibrates instantaneously between tissues. Thus the drug concentration–time profile shows a monophasic response (i.e. it is monoexponential; Figure 1.2a).

It is important to note that this does not imply that the drug concentration in plasma (C_p) is equal to the drug concentration in the tissues. However, changes in the plasma concentration quantitatively reflect changes in the tissues. The relationship described in Figure 1.2a can be plotted on a log C_p vs time graph (Figure 1.2b) and will then show a linear relation; this represents a one-compartment model.

Two-compartment model

The two-compartment model resolves the body into a central compartment and a peripheral compartment (see Figure 1.3). Although these compartments have no physiological or anatomical meaning, it is assumed that the central compartment comprises tissues that are highly perfused such as heart, lungs, kidneys, liver and brain. The peripheral compartment comprises less well-perfused tissues such as muscle, fat and skin.

A two-compartment model assumes that, following drug administration into the central compartment, the drug distributes between that compartment and the peripheral compartment. However, the drug does not achieve instantaneous distribution, i.e. equilibration, between the two compartments.

The drug concentration–time profile shows a curve (Figure 1.4a), but the log drug concentration–time plot shows a biphasic response

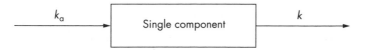

Figure 1.1 One-compartment model. k_a = absorption rate constant (h^{-1}), k = elimination rate constant (h^{-1}).

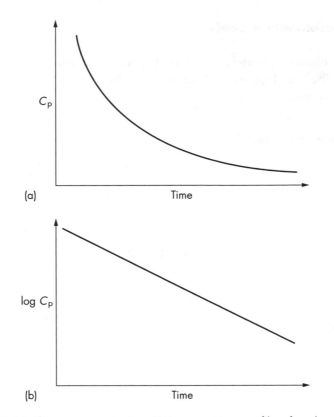

Figure 1.2 (a) Plasma concentration (C_p) versus time profile of a drug showing a one-compartment model. (b) Time profile of a one-compartment model showing log C_p versus time.

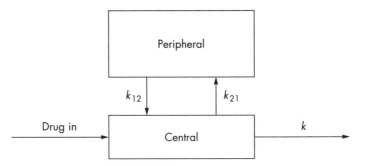

Figure 1.3 Two-compartment model. k_{12}, k_{21} and k are first-order rate constants: k_{12} = rate of transfer from central to peripheral compartment; k_{21} = rate of transfer from peripheral to central compartment; k = rate of elimination from central compartment.

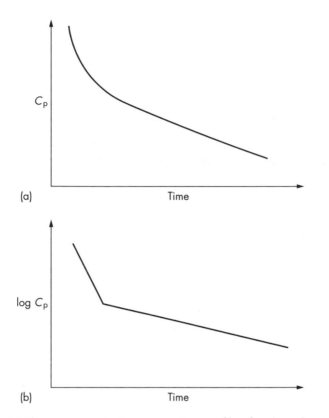

(a)   Time

(b)   Time

Figure 1.4 (a) Plasma concentration versus time profile of a drug showing a two-compartment model. (b) Time profile of a two-compartment model showing log C_p versus time.

(Figure 1.4b) and can be used to distinguish whether a drug shows a one- or two-compartment model.

Figure 1.4b shows a profile in which initially there is a rapid decline in the drug concentration owing to elimination from the central compartment and distribution to the peripheral compartment. Hence during this rapid initial phase the drug concentration will decline rapidly from the central compartment, rise to a maximum in the peripheral compartment, and then decline.

After a time interval (t), a distribution equilibrium is achieved between the central and peripheral compartments, and elimination of the drug is assumed to occur from the central compartment. As with the one-compartment model, all the rate processes are described by first-order reactions.

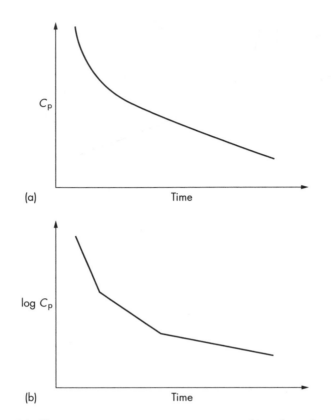

Figure 1.5 (a) Plasma concentration versus time profile of a drug showing multicompartment model. (b) Time profile of a multicompartment model showing log C_p versus time.

Multicompartment model

In this model the drug distributes into more than one compartment and the concentration–time profile shows more than one exponential (Figure 1.5a). Each exponential on the concentration–time profile describes a compartment. For example, gentamicin can be described by a three-compartment model following a single IV dose (see Figure 1.5b).

Pharmacokinetic parameters

This section describes various applications using the one-compartment open model system.

Elimination rate constant

Consider a single IV bolus injection of drug X (see Figure 1.2). As time proceeds, the amount of drug in the body is eliminated. Thus the rate of elimination can be described (assuming first-order elimination) as:

$$\frac{dX}{dt} = -kX$$

Hence

$$X = X_0 \exp(-kt)$$

where X = amount of drug X, X_0 = dose and k = first-order elimination rate constant.

Volume of distribution

The volume of distribution (V_d) has no direct physiological meaning; it is not a 'real' volume and is usually referred to as the *apparent volume of distribution*. It is defined as *that volume of plasma in which the total amount of drug in the body would be required to be dissolved in order to reflect the drug concentration attained in plasma.*

The body is not a homogeneous unit, even though a one-compartment model can be used to describe the plasma concentration–time profile of a number of drugs. It is important to realise that the concentration of the drug (C_p) in plasma is not necessarily the same in the liver, kidneys or other tissues.

Thus C_p in plasma does not equal C_p or amount of drug (X) in the kidney or C_p or amount of drug (X) in the liver or C_p or amount of drug (X) in tissues. However, changes in the drug concentration in plasma (C_p) are proportional to changes in the amount of drug (X) in the tissues. Since

$$C_p \text{ (plasma)} \propto C_p \text{ (tissues) i.e. } C_p \text{ (plasma)} \propto X \text{ (tissues)}$$

Then

$$C_p \text{ (plasma)} = V_d \times X \text{ (tissues)}$$

where V_d is the constant of proportionality and is referred to as the volume of distribution, which thus relates the total amount of drug in the body at any time to the corresponding plasma concentration. Thus

$$V_d = \frac{X}{C_p}$$

and V_d can be used to convert drug amount X to concentration. Since

$$X = X_0 \exp(-kt)$$

then

$$\frac{X}{V_d} = \frac{X_0 \exp(-kt)}{V_d}$$

Thus

$$C_{pt} = C_p^0 \exp(-kt)$$

This formula describes a monoexponential decay (see Figure 1.2), where C_{pt} = plasma concentration at any time t.

The curve can be converted to a linear form (Figure 1.6) using natural logarithms (ln):

$$\ln C_{pt} = \ln C_p^0 - kt$$

where the slope $= -k$, the elimination rate constant; and the y intercept $= \ln C_p^0$. Since

$$V_d = \frac{X}{C_p}$$

then at zero concentration (C_p^0), the amount administered is the dose, D, so that

$$C_p^0 = \frac{D}{V_d}$$

If the drug has a large V_d that does not equate to a real volume, e.g. total plasma volume, this suggests that the drug is highly distributed in tissues. On the other hand, if the V_d is similar to the total plasma volume this will suggest that the total amount of drug is poorly distributed and is mainly in the plasma.

Half-life

The time required to reduce the plasma concentration to one half its initial value is defined as the *half-life* ($t_{1/2}$).

Consider

$$\ln C_{pt} = \ln C_p^0 - kt$$

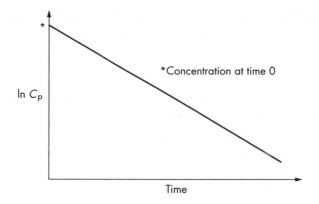

Figure 1.6 Ln C_p versus time profile.

Let C_p^0 decay to $C_p^0/2$ and solve for $t = t_{1/2}$:

$$\ln(C_p^0/2) = \ln C_p^0 - kt_{1/2}$$

Hence

$$kt_{1/2} = \ln C_p^0 - \ln(C_p^0/2)$$

and

$$t_{1/2} = \frac{(\ln 2)}{k}$$

$$t_{1/2} = \frac{0.693}{k}$$

This parameter is very useful for estimating how long it will take for levels to be reduced by half the original concentration. It can be used to estimate for how long a drug should be stopped if a patient has toxic drug levels, assuming the drug shows linear one-compartment pharmacokinetics.

Clearance

Drug clearance (CL) is defined as the volume of plasma in the vascular compartment cleared of drug per unit time by the processes of metabolism and excretion. Clearance for a drug is constant if the drug is eliminated by first-order kinetics. Drug can be cleared by renal excretion or by metabolism or both. With respect to the kidney and liver, etc., clearances are additive, that is:

$$CL_{total} = CL_{renal} + CL_{nonrenal}$$

Mathematically, clearance is the product of the first-order elimination rate constant (k) and the apparent volume of distribution (V_d). Thus

$$CL_{total} = k \times V_d$$

Hence the clearance is the elimination rate constant – i.e. the fractional rate of drug loss – from the volume of distribution.

Clearance is related to half-life by

$$t_{1/2} = \frac{0.693 \times V_d}{CL}$$

If a drug has a CL of 2 L/h, this tells you that 2 litres of the V_d is cleared of drug per hour. If the C_p is 10 mg/L, then 20 mg of drug is cleared per hour.

Pharmacokinetic applications

This section describes how pharmacokinetics can be used in clinical practice.

Single IV administration

Decay from a toxic level

For example, patient D has a potentially toxic digoxin level of 4.5 µg/L. Given that the half-life of digoxin in this patient is 60 h, and assuming that renal function is stable and absorption is complete, for how long should the drug be stopped to allow the level to fall to 1.5 µg/L?

(a) Calculate elimination rate constant (k):

$$k = \frac{0.693}{60}$$
$$= 0.0116 \text{ h}^{-1}$$

(b) Time for decay (t) from C_{p1} to C_{p2}

$$t = \frac{\ln C_{p1} - \ln C_{p2}}{k}$$
$$t = \frac{\ln 4.5 - \ln 1.5}{0.0116}$$
$$= 94.7 \text{ h}$$

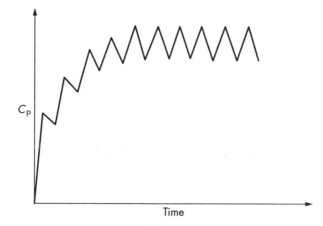

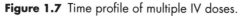

Figure 1.7 Time profile of multiple IV doses.

Hence

$$t = 4 \text{ days}$$

Multiple doses

Some drugs may be used clinically on a single-dose basis, although most drugs are administered continually over a period of time. When a drug is administered at a regular dosing interval (orally or IV), the drug accumulates in the body and the serum concentration will rise until steady-state conditions have been reached, assuming the drug is administered again before all of the previous dose has been eliminated (see Figure 1.7).

Steady state

Steady state occurs when the amount of drug administered (in a given time period) is equal to the amount of drug eliminated in that same period. At steady state the plasma concentrations of the drug (C_p^{ss}) at any time during any dosing interval, as well as the peak and trough, are similar. The time to reach steady-state concentrations is dependent on the half-life of the drug under consideration.

Effect of dose

The higher the dose, the higher the steady-state levels, but the time to achieve steady-state levels is independent of dose (see Figure 1.8). Note that the fluctuations in $C_{p\,max}$ and $C_{p\,min}$ are greatest with higher doses.

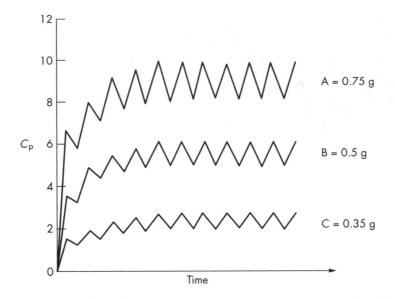

Figure 1.8 Time profiles of multiple IV doses – reaching steady state using different doses.

Effect of dosing interval

Consider a drug having a half-life of 3 h. When the dosing interval, τ, is less than the half-life, $t_{1/2}$, greater accumulation occurs, i.e. higher steady-state levels are higher and there is less fluctuation in $C_{p\,max}$ and $C_{p\,min}$ (see Figure 1.9, curve A). When $\tau > t_{1/2}$, then a lower accumulation occurs with greater fluctuation in $C_{p\,max}$ and $C_{p\,min}$ (see Figure 1.9, curve C).

If the dosing interval is much greater than the half-life of the drug, then $C_{p\,min}$ approaches zero. Under these conditions no accumulation will occur and the plasma concentration–time profile will be the result of administration of a series of single doses.

Time to reach steady state

For a drug with one-compartment characteristics, the time to reach steady state is independent of the dose, the number of doses administered, and the dosing interval, but it is directly proportional to the half-life.

Prior to steady state

As an example, estimate the plasma concentration 12 h after therapy commences with drug A given 500 mg three times a day.

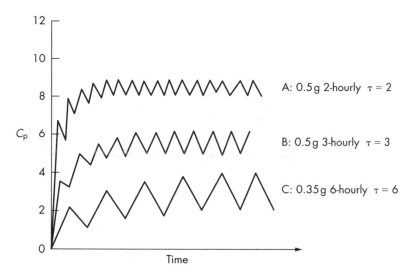

Figure 1.9 Time profiles of multiple IV doses – reaching steady state using different dosing intervals.

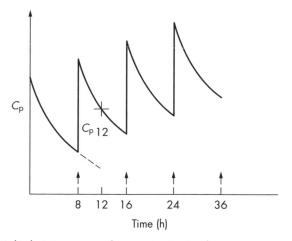

Figure 1.10 Multiple intravenous doses prior to steady state.

Consider each dose as independent and calculate the contribution of each dose to the plasma level at 12 h post dose (see Figure 1.10).

From the first dose:

$$C_{p1} = C_p^0 \exp(-k \times 12)$$

From the second dose:

$$C_{p2} = C_p^0 \exp(-k \times 4)$$

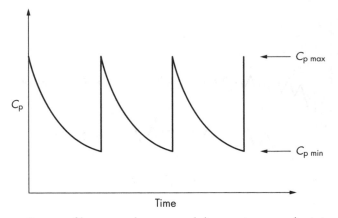

Figure 1.11 Time profile at steady state and the maximum and minimum plasma concentration within a dosage interval.

Thus, total C_{pt} at 12 h is

$$C_{pt} = C_p^0 \exp(-k \times 12) + C_p^0 \exp(-k \times 4)$$

Remember that $C_p^0 = D/V_d$.

This method uses the principle of superposition. The following equation can be used to simplify the process of calculating the value of C_p at any time t after the nth dose:

$$C_{pt} = \frac{D \times [\exp(-kn\tau) \times [\exp(-kt)]}{V_d \times [1 - \exp(-k\tau)]}$$

where n = number of doses, τ = dosing interval and t = time after the nth dose.

At steady state

To describe the plasma concentration (C_p) at any time (t) within a dosing interval (τ) at steady state (see Figure 1.11):

$$C_{pt} = \frac{D \times [\exp(-kt)]}{V_d \times [1 - \exp(-k\tau)]}$$

Remember that $C_p^0 = D/V_d$. Alternatively, for some drugs it is important to consider the salt factor (S). Hence, if applicable, $C_p^0 = SD/V_d$ and:

$$C_{pt} = \frac{S \times D \times [\exp(-kt)]}{V_d \times [1 - \exp(-k\tau)]}$$

To describe the maximum plasma concentration at steady state (i.e. $t = 0$ and $\exp(-kt) = 1$):

$$C_{p\,max} = \frac{D \times 1}{V_d \times [1 - \exp(-k\tau)]}$$

To describe the minimum plasma concentration at steady state (i.e. $t = \tau$):

$$C_{p\,min} = \frac{D \times [\exp(-k\tau)]}{V_d \times [1 - \exp(-k\tau)]}$$

To describe the average steady-state concentration, C_p^{ss} (this notation will be used throughout the book):

$$C_p^{ss} = \frac{D}{CL \times \tau} \quad \text{or} \quad C_p^{ss} = \frac{S \times D}{CL \times \tau}$$

Since

$$t_{1/2} = \frac{0.693 \times V_d}{CL}$$

then

$$C_p^{ss} = \frac{1.44 \times D \times t_{1/2}}{V_d \times \tau}$$

Steady state from first principles

At steady state the rate of drug administration is equal to the rate of drug elimination. Mathematically the rate of drug administration can be stated in terms of the dose (D) and dosing interval (τ). It is always important to include the salt factor (S) and the bioavailability (F). The rate of drug elimination will be the clearance of the plasma concentration at steady state:

$$\text{Rate of drug administration} = \frac{S \times F \times D}{\tau}$$

$$\text{Rate of drug elimination} = CL \times C_p^{ss}$$

At steady state:

$$\frac{S \times F \times D}{\tau} = CL \times C_p^{ss}$$

Table 1.2 In practice, steady state is assumed to be reached in 5 half-lives. If we assume a patient is receiving 100-mg doses and half the total amount is eliminated at each half life, the table shows the time to reach steady-state concentration in the body

Dose (mg)	Amount in the body (mg)	Amount eliminated (mg)	Number of half lives
100	100	50	1
100	150	75	2
100	175	87.5	3
100	187.5	93.75	4
100	197.5	98.75	5
100	198.75	99.37	6
100	199.37[a]	99.68	7

[a] Continuing at this rate of dosage, the amount of drug in the body will remain the same.

Rearranging the equation:

$$C_p^{ss} = \frac{S \times F \times D}{CL \times \tau}$$

In practice, steady state is assumed to be reached in 4–5 half-lives. If we assume that a patient is receiving a 100-mg dose and half the total amount is eliminated at each half-life, Table 1.2 shows the time to reach a steady-state concentration in the body.

Intravenous infusion

Some drugs are administered as an intravenous infusion rather than as an intravenous bolus. To describe the time course of the drug in plasma during the infusion prior to steady state (see Figure 1.12), one can use:

$$C_{pt} = \frac{R[1 - \exp(-kt)]}{CL}$$

where

$$R = \frac{D}{\tau}$$

or

$$R = \frac{S \times D}{\tau}$$

if a salt of the drug is given.

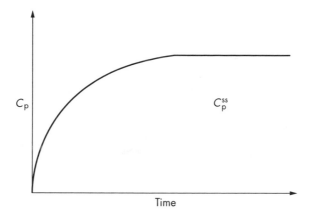

Figure 1.12 Time profile after IV infusion.

Following a continuous infusion, the plasma concentrations will increase with time until the rate of elimination (rate out) equals the rate of infusion (rate in) and will then remain constant. The plateau concentration, i.e. C_p^{ss}, is the steady-state concentration. Steady state will be achieved in 4–5 times the $t_{1/2}$. If one considers the previous equation, which describes the plasma concentration during the infusion prior to steady state, then at steady state,

$$\exp(-kt) = 0$$

As rate in = rate out at steady state,

$$R = CL \times C_p^{ss}$$

$$C_p^{ss} = \frac{D}{\tau \times CL}$$

where $R = D/\tau$ = infusion rate (dose/h).

When a constant infusion is stopped, the drug concentrations in the plasma decline in an exponential manner, as illustrated in Figure 1.13.

To estimate the plasma concentration, C_p' at t' one must describe the decay of C_p^{ss} at time t to C_p' at time t'. Thus, from the above:

$$C_p^{ss} = \frac{D}{\tau \times CL}$$

To describe the decay of C_p from t to t', one uses the single-dose IV bolus equation

$$C_{pt} = C_p^0[\exp(-kt)]$$

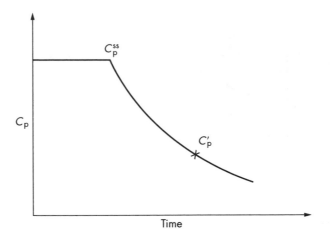

Figure 1.13 Profile following discontinuation of an infusion.

Since C_p^0 is C_p^{ss}, then from the above,

$$C_p' = \frac{D \, \exp[-k(t' - t)]}{\tau \times CL}$$

Loading dose

The time required to obtain steady-state plasma levels by IV infusion will be long if a drug has a long half-life. It is, therefore, useful in such cases to administer an intravenous loading dose to attain the desired drug concentration immediately and then attempt to maintain this concentration by a continuous infusion.

To estimate the loading dose (LD), where C_p^{ss} is the final desired concentration, use

$$LD = V_d \times C_p^{ss}$$

If the patient has already received the drug, then the loading dose should be adjusted accordingly:

$$LD = V_d \times (C_p^{ss} - C_p^{initial})$$

or

$$LD = \frac{V_d \times (C_p^{ss} - C_p^{initial})}{S}$$

if the salt of the drug (salt factor S) is used.

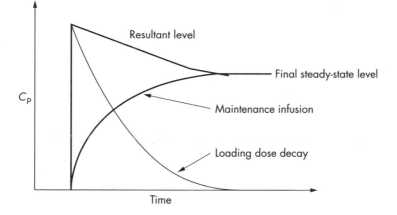

Figure 1.14 Profile following a loading dose and maintenance infusion.

Now consider the plasma concentration–time profile following a loading dose and maintenance infusion (see Figure 1.14). The equation to describe the time course of the plasma concentrations of drug following simultaneous administration of an IV loading dose (LD) and initiation of infusion (D) is the sum of the two equations describing these two processes individually:

$$C_p = \frac{LD \; exp(-kt)}{V_d} + \frac{D[1 - exp(-kt)]}{\tau \times CL}$$

The final plasma concentration achieved is not the 'true' steady-state concentration, since that will still require about 4 half-lives to be reached, but depending on the accuracy of the loading dose it will be fairly close. However, this regimen allows the concentration somewhere near steady state to be achieved more rapidly. If the salt is used:

$$C_p = \frac{S \times LD \; exp(-kt)}{V_d} + \frac{S \times D[1 - exp(-kt)]}{\tau \times CL}$$

Single oral dose

The plasma concentration–time profile of a large number of drugs can be described by a one-compartment model with first-order absorption and elimination.

Consider the concentration versus time profile following a single oral dose (Figure 1.15). Assuming first-order absorption and first-order

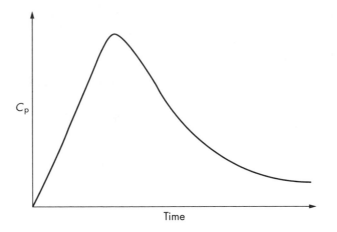

Figure 1.15 Single oral dose profile.

elimination, the rate of change of amount of drug (X) in the body is described by:

$$\frac{dX}{dt} = k_a X_a - kX$$

where k_a = absorption rate constant; k = elimination rate constant; X = amount of drug in the body; and X_a = amount of drug at the absorption site (X_0 if all is available). Following integration:

$$X = \frac{X_0\, k_a\, [\exp(-kt) - \exp(-k_a t)]}{k_a - k}$$

To convert X to C_p one uses the apparent volume of distribution (V_d). Furthermore, following oral administration, the bioavailability (F) and salt factor (S) (see below) must be considered.

Fractional bioavailability, F

F is the fraction of an oral dose that reaches the systemic circulation, which following oral administration may be less than 100%. Thus, if $F = 0.5$ then 50% of the drug is absorbed. Parenteral dosage forms (IM and IV) assume a bioavailability of 100%, and so $F = 1$; it is therefore not considered and is omitted from calculations.

If the loading dose is to be administered orally, then the bioavailability term (F) needs to be introduced. Thus:

$$LD = \frac{V_d \times C_p}{F}$$

Salt factor, S

S is the fraction of the administered dose, which may be in the form of an ester or salt, that is the active drug. Aminophylline is the ethylenediamine salt of theophylline, and S is 0.79. Thus 1 g aminophylline is equivalent to 790 mg theophylline.

Accordingly, S needs to be incorporated along with F into the oral loading dose equation and the equation that describes the plasma concentration C_p at any time t following a single oral dose. Thus,

$$LD = \frac{V_d \times C_p}{S \times F}$$

and

$$C_{pt} = \frac{SFD}{V_d} \times \frac{k_a[\exp(-kt) - \exp(-k_a t)]}{k_a - k}$$

N.B. The S factor may need to be considered during IV infusion administration.

Multiple oral dosing

Prior to steady state

Consider a patient on medication prescribed three times a day. The profile shown in Figure 1.16 shows the administration of three doses. If we consider a time 28 h into therapy, all three doses would have been administered.

To calculate C_p at 28 h post dose, use the single oral dose equation and consider the contributions of each dose:

Contribution from dose 1; $t_1 = 28$ h:

$$C_{p1} = \frac{SFD}{V_d} \times \frac{k_a[\exp(-kt_1) - \exp(-k_a t_1)]}{k_a - k}$$

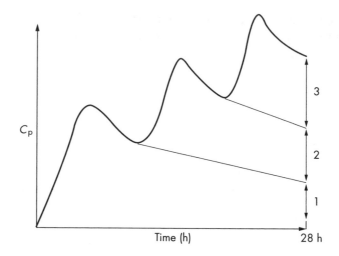

Figure 1.16 Multiple dosing prior to steady state.

Contribution from dose 2, $t_2 = 18$ h:

$$C_{p2} = \frac{SFD}{V_d} \times \frac{k_a[\exp(-kt_2) - \exp(-k_a t_2)]}{k_a - k}$$

Contribution from dose 3; $t_3 = 8$ h:

$$C_{p3} = \frac{SFD}{V_d} \times \frac{k_a[\exp(-kt_3) - \exp(-k_a t_3)]}{k_a - k}$$

Thus,

$$C_{p28h} = C_{p1} + C_{p2} + C_{p3}$$

The above method uses the principle of superposition to calculate the C_p at any time t after the nth dose. The following equation can simplify the process.

$$C_{pt} = \frac{SFDk_a}{V_d(k_a - k)} \times \left\{ \frac{[1 - \exp(-nk\tau)](\exp(-kt))}{1 - \exp(-k\tau)} \right.$$

$$\left. - \frac{[1 - \exp(-nk_a\tau)](\exp(-k_a t))}{1 - \exp(-k_a\tau)} \right\}$$

where n = number of doses, τ = dosage interval and t = time after the nth dose.

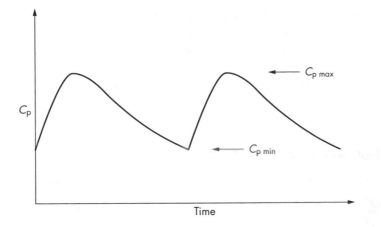

Figure 1.17 Multiple dosing at steady state.

At steady state

At steady state the plasma concentration–time profile can be described by

$$C_{pt} = \frac{SFDk_a}{V_d(k_a - k)} \times \left\{ \frac{\exp(-kt)}{1 - \exp(-k\tau)} - \frac{\exp(-k_a t)}{1 - \exp(-k_a \tau)} \right\}$$

The plasma concentration at steady state fluctuates between a maximum ($C_{p\ max}$) and a minimum ($C_{p\ min}$) concentration, within a dose interval (see Figure 1.17).

To estimate $C_{p\ max}$, one first needs to estimate time to peak (t_{pk}):

$$t_{pk} = \frac{1}{k_a - k} \times \ln \frac{k_a[1 - \exp(-k\tau)]}{k[1 - e(-k_a \tau)]}$$

Note that t_{pk} is independent of the dose administered. Thus,

$$C_{p\ max} = \frac{SFDk_a}{V_d(k_a - k)} \times \left\{ \frac{\exp(-kt_{pk})}{1 - \exp(-k\tau)} - \frac{\exp(-k_a t_{pk})}{1 - \exp(-k_a \tau)} \right\}$$

The minimum plasma concentration at steady state occurs just before the next dose, i.e., when $t = \tau$. So

$$C_{p\ min} = \frac{SFDk_a}{V_d(k_a - k)} \times \left\{ \frac{\exp(-k\tau)}{1 - \exp(-k\tau)} - \frac{\exp(-k_a \tau)}{1 - \exp(-k_a \tau)} \right\}$$

When using these formulae, individual values should be calculated, since they are often used more than once.

When the half-life of a drug is long, the fluctuations between the peak and trough are small, and the equation derived above under Intravenous infusion (p. 18) can be used to describe the average steady-state concentration:

$$C_p^{ss} = \frac{D}{T \times CL}$$

Clinical case studies

CASE STUDY 1.1   Multiple IV bolus

Patient D receives Drug Code XR2, 100 mg every 8 h. At steady state, two plasma concentrations are measured:

    Sample 1 is taken at 1 h post dose: Conc = 9.6 mg/L
    Sample 2 is taken pre dose: Conc = 2.9 mg/L
    See Figure 1.18

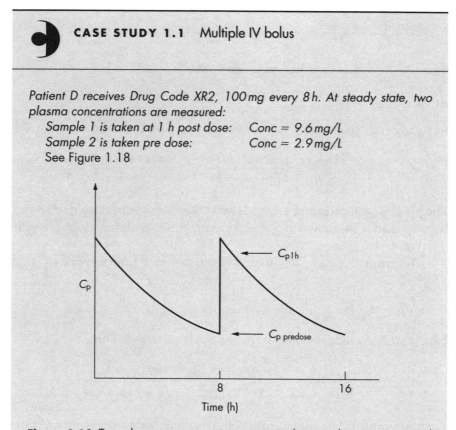

Figure 1.18 Two plasma concentrations measured at steady state, $C_{p\ 1h}$ and $C_{p\ predose}$.

Since the samples were taken at steady state, the pre-dose sample represents the trough concentration. $C_{p\ max}$, C_{pt} and $C_{p\ min}$ will be the same within each dosing interval.

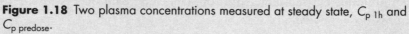

Calculate the elimination rate constant (k)

$$k = \frac{\ln\ C_{p1} - \ln\ C_{p2}}{t_2 - t_1}$$

Now C_{p1} is 9.6 mg/L and C_{p2} is 2.9 mg/L, and sample times are 1 h and 8 h (extrapolated). Thus

$$t_2 - t_1 = 7\,h$$

So

$$k = \frac{\ln 9.6 - \ln 2.9}{7} = \frac{1.197}{7}$$

$$k = 0.171 h^{-1}$$

and the half-life ($t_{1/2}$) is

$$t_{1/2} = \frac{0.693}{0.171} = 4.1\,h$$

Calculate the volume of distribution (V_d)
The volume can be calculated from either the 1 h post- or pre-dose samples.

From the 1 h post-dose sample
The following equation describes the plasma concentration 1 h post dose at steady state:

$$C_{p1} = \frac{D \times \exp(-kt)}{V_d[1 - \exp(-k\tau)]}$$

Thus

$$V_d = \frac{D \times \exp(-kt)}{C_{p1}[1 - \exp(-k\tau)]}$$

$$V_d = \frac{100\ e^{-0.1710 \times 1}}{9.6(1 - e^{-0.1710 \times 8})}$$

$$= \frac{100 \times 0.8428}{9.6 \times 0.7454}$$

$$= 11.8\ L$$

$\rightarrow$

CASE STUDY 1.1 (continued)

From the pre-dose sample
The following equation describes $C_{p,min}$ at steady state:

$$C_{p\,min} = \frac{D \times exp(-k\tau)}{V_d[1 - exp(-k\tau)]}$$

$$V_d = \frac{D \times exp(-k\tau)}{C_{p\,min}[1 - exp(-k\tau)]}$$

$$V_d = \frac{100\,e^{-0.1710\times8}}{2.9(1 - e^{-0.1710\times8})}$$

$$= \frac{100 \times 0.2546}{2.9 \times 0.7454}$$

$$= 11.8\,L$$

Calculate clearance

$$CL = k \times V_d$$
$$= 0.171 \times 11.8$$
$$= 2.02\,L/h$$

Individualised pharmacokinetic parameters
The patient's individual parameters are as follows:
Elimination rate constant (k) $0.171\,h^{-1}$
Volume of distribution (V_d) $11.8\,L$
Clearance (CL) $2.02\,L/h$
Half-life ($t_{1/2}$) $4.1\,h$
Time to steady state (t_{ss}) $18.5\,h$

CASE STUDY 1.2   Oral dose

Patient H, aged 40 years and weighing 60 kg, receives an oral dose of Drug Code XR4, 500 mg every 12 h. The patient is at steady state. A plasma level is measured at 10 h post dose and is reported to be 18.2 mg/L.

$\rightarrow$

Assume one-compartment kinetics, all doses were given and $F = 1$. Estimate patient H's individualised pharmacokinetic data.
Data given:

$V_d = 0.4 \, \text{L/kg}$

$CL = 0.05 \, \text{L/h/kg}$

$k_a = 0.4 \, \text{h}^{-1}$

$S = 1$

Use population data to obtain starting parameters

$V_d = 0.4 \times 60 = 24 \, \text{L}$

$CL = 0.05 \times 60 = 3.0 \, \text{L/h}$

$k = 0.125 \, \text{h}^{-1}$

$t_{1/2} = 5.5 \, \text{h}$

Estimate C_{pt} at sampling time (i.e. $C_{p\,predicted}$), $t = 10 \, \text{h}$

$$C_{pt} = \frac{SFDk_a}{[V_d(k_a - k)]} \times \frac{\exp(-kt)}{1 - \exp(-k\tau)} \times \frac{\exp(-k_a t)}{1 - \exp(-k_a \tau)}$$

Now

$$SFDk_a = 1 \times 1 \times 500 \times 0.4$$

and

$$V_d(k_a - k) = 24(0.4 - 0.125)$$

and the exponential part is

$$\frac{(e^{-0.125 \times 10})}{(1 - e^{-0.125 \times 12})} - \frac{(e^{-0.4 \times 10})}{(1 - e^{-0.4 \times 12})}$$

Thus

$$C_{pt} = \frac{200}{6.6} \left(\frac{0.2865}{0.7768} - \frac{0.0183}{0.9918} \right)$$

$$= 10.6 \, \text{mg/L}$$

$\rightarrow$

> **CASE STUDY 1.2** (continued)

Compare $C_{p\,predicted}$ with $C_{p\,measured}$
Assess whether the patient is 'clearing' the drug faster or slower than the initial population data estimate. Assume the volume of distribution is fixed. From the data, the predicted concentration, 10.6 mg/L, when compared with the measured value of 8.2 mg/L, does suggest that the patient's clearance is faster than population data.

Alter k accordingly by the process of iteration
Let $k = 0.10\,h^{-1}$. Thus

$$CL = 2.4\,L/h$$

Predict C_{pt} at 10 h post dose using the above information; k_a remains the same:

$$V_d(k_a - k) = 24(0.4 - 0.10)$$

and the exponential part is

$$\frac{e^{-0.10\times10}}{1 - e^{-0.4\times10}} - \frac{e^{-0.10\times12}}{e^{-0.4\times12}}$$

Thus

$$C_{p10h} = 14.1\,mg/L$$

Still $C_{p\,predicted}$ is less than $C_{p\,measured}$.
Let $k = 0.08\,h^{-1}$. Thus

$$CL = 1.92\,L/h$$

Predict C_{pt} at 10 h post dose:

$$V_d(k_a - k) = 24(0.4 - 0.08)$$

and the exponential part is

$$\frac{e^{-0.08\times10}}{1 - e^{-0.4\times12}} - \frac{e^{-0.08\times10}}{1 - e^{-0.4\times12}}$$

Thus

$$C_{p10h} = 18.4\,mg/L$$

Now $C_{p\,predicted}$ is very close to $C_{p\,measured}$.

$\longrightarrow$

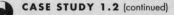

CASE STUDY 1.2 (continued)

Summary

k (h^{-1})	CL (L/h)	$C_{p\ predicted}$ (mg/L)
0.125	3.0	10.6
0.10	2.4	14.1
0.08	1.92	18.4

Hence using $k = 0.08\,h^{-1}$ the predicted concentration is 18.4 mg/L, which is similar to the observed concentration of 18.2 mg/L.

The patient's observed pharmacokinetic parameters

$$CL = 1.92\,L/h$$
$$V_d = 24\,L$$
$$k = 0.08\,h^{-1}$$
$$t = 8.6\,h$$

Note that the volume of distribution of 0.4 L/kg is assumed to be constant.

Assessment of individualised data

In practice the glossary of equations described (p. 37) can be used to simulate plasma concentration vs time profiles for a dosage regimen using different routes of administration. The important issue is to utilise mean pharmacokinetics parameters derived from research that match the clinical and demographic data of the patient. Basic data can be obtained from original research papers or from the pharmaceutical industry for the specific drug. Where possible the equations that describe the average steady state concentration (C_p^{ss}) can be used to estimate the levels in the patient. Pharmacokinetic interpretation and estimation of a patient's actual pharmacokinetic data, e.g. CL, relies on plasma concentrations measured at a specific time following drug administration where this depicts the average plasma concentration.

The basic questions to be asked when determining which set of equations to use follows the algorithm described in Figure 1.22.

To determine whether the data are acceptable, see monographs on individual drugs because, for TDM, the individual parameters must be

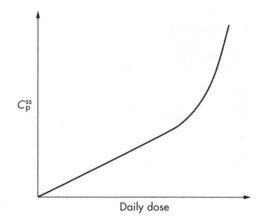

Figure 1.19 C_p^{ss} profile following different doses of phenytoin.

interpreted in light of the patient's dosage details, clinical status, and so on (see individual drug monographs in the following chapters).

Nonlinear pharmacokinetics: Basic parameters

Drugs such as phenytoin will show nonlinear drug handing. The process of metabolism are nonlinear and the rate of metabolism shows zero order. In practice, Michaelis–Menten pharmacokinetics are applied, and the equations are summarised below.

If a patient receives different doses of phenytoin, e.g. 200 mg/day, 250 mg/day, 300 mg/day or 400 mg/day, the steady-state plasma concentration varies exponentially with time; that is, a small change in the total daily dose of phenytoin shows a disproportionate increase in the steady-state concentration (C_p^{ss}) (Figure 1.19).

Figure 1.20 describes the profile of the rate of metabolism of phenytoin given at different dosages. As the dose of phenytoin increases, the rate of elimination increases until it reaches a plateau where the rate of elimination is constant despite increases in the total daily dose of the drug. The profile can be described as follows.
Rate of elimination:

$$\frac{-dX}{dt} = \frac{V_m \times C_p^{ss}}{K_m + C_p^{ss}}$$

Hence the model that appears to fit the pattern for the metabolic elimination of phenytoin is not linear and is the one proposed by Michaelis and

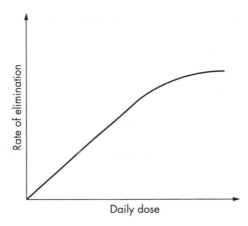

Figure 1.20 Profile of elimination following phenytoin administration.

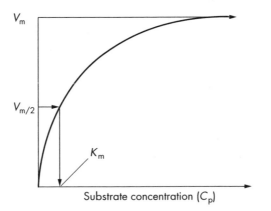

Figure 1.21 Relationship between rate of metabolism (V) versus substrate concentration (C_p) for a drug showing nonlinear pharmacokinetics.

Menten. The velocity (V) or rate at which an enzyme can metabolise a substrate (C_p) can be described by the following equation:

$$V = -\frac{V_m \times C_p}{K_m + C_p}$$

where V is the rate of metabolism, V_m (sometimes referred to as V_{max}) is the maximum rate of metabolism and K_m is the substrate concentration (C_p) at which V will be half V_m, i.e. when half the total enzyme is complexed with the substrate. (See Figure 1.21.)

At steady state we know that the rate of administration is equal to the rate of elimination; hence, in the clinical situation, the daily dose (R, or D) is substituted for velocity (V), and the steady-state phenytoin concentration (C_p^{ss}) is substituted for substrate concentration (S). Further equations can be described for steady-state concentrations.

At steady state the rate of administration is equal to the rate of elimination. The rate of administration can be expressed as SFD/τ where D/τ can equal R. Hence

$$RSF = \frac{V_m \times C_p^{ss}}{K_m + C_p^{ss}}$$

V_m is the maximum metabolic capacity, i.e. the total amount of drug that can be eliminated at saturation. K_m is the Michaelis constant, which by definition is the concentration at which the metabolism is operating at half the maximum capacity.

All drugs will show nonlinear handling if they are administered in high enough doses. However, only a small number of drugs show nonlinear handling at the doses used clinically.

Whether a drug will show linear or nonlinear drug handling in therapeutic doses depends on the drug's Michaelis constant K_m. For example, consider a drug that has a K_m that is much greater then C_p^{ss}, i.e. the plasma levels seen with normal therapeutic doses of the drug. The rate of elimination can be described as

$$\frac{-dX}{dt} = \frac{V_m \times C_p^{ss}}{K_m + C_p^{ss}}$$

Since K_m is much more than C_p^{ss}, the equation simplifies to

$$\frac{-dX}{dt} = \frac{V_m \times C_p^{ss}}{K_m}$$

Since V_m and K_m are constants, this now represents a first-order process.

In another simulation a drug has a K_m that is much less than C_p^{ss}, i.e. the plasma levels seen with normal therapeutic doses of the drug.

$$\frac{-dX}{dt} = \frac{V_m \times C_p^{ss}}{K_m + C_p^{ss}}$$

Since K_m is much less than C_p^{ss}, the equation simplifies to

$$\frac{-dX}{dt} = V_m$$

Since V_m is a constant, this now represents a zero-order process.

Hence, the relationship between the Michaelis constant (K_m) of the drug and the plasma levels of the drug normally achieved with therapeutic dosages will determine whether the drug will show linear first-order or zero-order saturation pharmacokinetics.

Practical clinical use of nonlinear equations

$$R \times F \times S = \frac{V_m \times C_p^{ss}}{K_m + C_p^{ss}}$$

The above equation can be used

- To calculate predicted C_p^{ss} from a given dosage regimen, to estimate the patient's V_m using population K_m values.
- To describe the relationship between the total daily dose R (mg/day) and the steady-state serum concentration.

$$C_p^{ss} = \frac{K_m \times (R \times F \times S)}{V_m - (R \times F \times S)}$$

$$R \times F \times S = \frac{(V_m - K_m) \times R}{C_p^{ss}}$$

$$C_p^{ss} = \frac{(V_m \times C_p^{ss}) - K_m}{R \times F \times S}$$

or

$$C_p^{ss} = \frac{(D_{max} \times C_p^{ss}) - K_m}{D}$$

N.B. The last three equations are linear relationships.

Clearance (CL) is the parameter that relates the rate of elimination to the plasma concentration. Since $CL = R/C_p^{ss}$,

$$CL = \frac{V_m}{K_m + C_p^{ss}}$$

And since apparent $t_{1/2} = (0.693 \times V_d)/CL$,

$$t_{1/2} = \frac{0.693 \times V_d(K_m + C_p^{ss})}{V_m}$$

From the above equations, it can be noted that the clearance and half-life will alter depending on the steady-state concentration. Thus V_m and K_m should be used to describe the kinetics of phenytoin and not clearance and half-life.

Toxic drug levels

For the decay of a toxic plasma concentration (C_p') to a desired plasma concentration (C_p):

$$C_{pt\ decay}' = \frac{(K_m \times \ln(C_p'/C_p)) + (C_p' - C_p)}{V_m/V_d}$$

where t decay = time (days) to allow C_p' to fall to C_p.

Phenytoin serum levels in the presence of altered plasma protein binding

To calculate a 'corrected' C_p^{ss} for a patient with a low serum albumin:

$$C_{p\ adjusted} = \frac{C_p^*}{(1 - \alpha)(P'/P) + \alpha}$$

where $C_{p\ adjusted}$ = plasma concentration that would be expected if the patient had a normal serum albumin; C_p^* = steady-state serum level observed; P' = serum albumin concentration observed; P = 'normal' serum albumin concentration (40 g/L); α = phenytoin free fraction (0.1).

To calculate a 'corrected' C_p^{ss} for a patient with both uraemia and hypoalbuminaemia:

$$C_{p\ adjusted} = \frac{C_p^*}{(1 - \alpha)(0.44\ P'/P) + \alpha}$$

where 0.44 is an empirical adjustment factor and $\alpha = 0.2$.

Chapter 10 on antiepileptics describes the clinical use of the above equations.

Glossary of pharmacokinetic equations and their application in clinical practice

$$C_p^0 = \frac{S \times F \times D}{V_d} \tag{1}$$

$$t_{1/2} = \frac{0.693}{k} \tag{2}$$

$$CL = k \times V_d \tag{3}$$

Single IV bolus injection

$$C_{pt} = C_p^0 \exp(-kt) \tag{4}$$

Single oral dose

Equation to describe plasma concentration at any time (t) after a single oral dose:

$$C_{pt} = C_p^0 \frac{k_a}{k_a - k} [\exp(-kt) - \exp(-k_a t)] \tag{5}$$

Multiple IV bolus injections

Equations to describe the concentration at any time within a dosing interval:

$$C_{pt}^{ss} = C_p^0 \left[\frac{\exp(-kt)}{1 - \exp(-k\tau)} \right] \tag{6a}$$

$$C_{p\,max}^{ss} = C_p^0 \left[\frac{1}{1 - \exp(-k\tau)} \right] \tag{6b}$$

$$C_{p\,min}^{ss} = C_p^0 \left[\frac{\exp(-k\tau)}{1 - \exp(-k\tau)} \right] \tag{6c}$$

IV infusion prior to steady state

$$C_{pt} = \frac{D \times S}{\tau \times CL} [1 - \exp(-kt)] \tag{7}$$

IV infusion at steady state

$$C_p^{ss} = \frac{D \times S}{\tau \times CL} \tag{8}$$

Multiple oral dosing at steady state

Equation to describe the concentration at any time (t) within a dosing interval, at steady state:

$$C_p^{ss} = C_p^0 \frac{k_a}{k_a - k} \left[\frac{\exp(-kt)}{1 - \exp(-k\tau)} - \frac{\exp(-k_a t)}{1 - \exp(-k_a\tau)} \right] \tag{9}$$

The maximum concentration is given by:

$$C_{p\,max}^{ss} = C_p^0 \frac{k_a}{k_a - k} \left[\frac{\exp(-kt_{max}^{ss})}{1 - \exp(-k\tau)} - \frac{\exp(-k_a t_{max}^{ss})}{1 - \exp(-k_a\tau)} \right] \tag{10}$$

The time at which the maximum concentration occurs is given by:

$$t_{max}^{ss} = \frac{1}{k_a - k} \ln \left\{ \frac{k_a[1 - \exp(-k\tau)]}{k[1 - \exp(-k_a\tau)]} \right\} \tag{11}$$

The minimum concentration is given by:

$$C_{p\,min}^{ss} = C_p^0 \frac{k_a}{k_a - k} \left[\frac{\exp(-k\tau)}{1 - \exp(-k\tau)} - \frac{\exp(-k_a\tau)}{1 - \exp(-k_a\tau)} \right] \tag{12}$$

Loading doses

$$LD = \frac{V_d \times C_p}{S \times F} \tag{13}$$

$$LD = \frac{V_d(C_{p\,desired} - C_{p\,observed})}{S \times F} \tag{14}$$

The average steady state concentration (C_p^{ss}) can be described by:

$$C_p^{ss} = \frac{S \times F \times D}{CL \times \tau} \tag{15}$$

Toxic level decay for drugs that show first-order elimination

$$\text{Time for decay} = \frac{\ln C_{p1} - \ln C_{p2}}{k} \tag{16}$$

Where C_{p1} = toxic plasma level and C_{p2} = desired plasma level.

Nonlinear pharmacokinetic equations

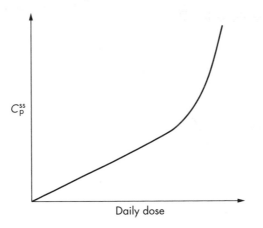

Figure 1.19 C_p^{ss} profile following different doses of phenytoin.

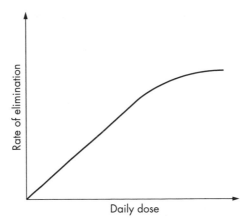

Figure 1.20 Profile of elimination following phenytoin administration.

Pharmacokinetic model

The model that appears to fit the pattern for the metabolic elimination of phenytoin is not linear and is the one proposed by Michaelis and

Menten. The velocity (V) or rate at which an enzyme can metabolise a substrate (C_p) can be described by the following equation:

$$V = \frac{V_m \times C_p}{K_m + C_p} \qquad (17)$$

where V is the rate of metabolism and V_m (sometimes referred to as V_{max}) is the maximum rate of metabolism and K_m is the substrate concentration at which V will be half V_m, i.e. when half the total enzyme is complexed with the substrate.

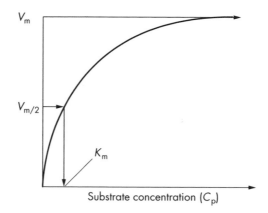

Figure 1.21 Relationship between rate of metabolism (V) versus substrate concentration (C_p) for a drug showing nonlinear pharmacokinetics.

When equation (18) is used in the clinical situation, the daily dose (R, or D) is substituted for velocity (V), and the steady-state phenytoin concentration (C_p^{ss}) is substituted for substrate concentration. Expressions can then be derived for steady state concentrations.

$$R \times F \times S = \frac{V_m \times C_p^{ss}}{K_m + C_p^{ss}} \qquad (18)$$

$$C_p^{ss} = \frac{K_m \times (R \times F \times S)}{V_m - (R \times F \times S)} \qquad (19)$$

$$R \times F \times S = \frac{(V_m - K_m) \times R}{C_p^{ss}} \qquad (20)$$

$$C_p^{ss} = \frac{(V_m \times C_p^{ss}) - K_m}{R \times F \times S} \qquad (21)$$

or

$$C_p^{ss} = \frac{(D_{max} \times C_p^{ss}) - K_m}{D} \tag{22}$$

Toxic drug levels

For the decay of a toxic plasma concentration (C_p') to a desired plasma concentration (C_p):

$$C_{pt\ decay}' = \frac{(K_m \times \ln(C_p'/C_p)) + (C_p' - C_p)}{V_m/V_d} \tag{23}$$

where t decay = time (days) to allow C_p' to fall to C_p.

Phenytoin serum levels in the presence of altered plasma protein binding

To calculate a 'corrected' C_p^{ss} or a patient with a low serum albumin:

$$C_{p\ adjusted} = \frac{C_p^*}{(1 - \alpha)(P'/P) + \alpha} \tag{24}$$

where $C_{p\ adjusted}$ = plasma concentration that would be expected if the patient had a normal serum albumin; C_p^* = steady-state serum level observed; P' = serum albumin concentration observed; P = 'normal' serum albumin concentration (40 g/L); α = phenytoin free fraction (0.1).

To calculate a 'corrected' C_p^{ss} for a patient with both uraemia and hypoalbuminaemia:

$$C_{p\ adjusted} = \frac{C_p^*}{(1 - \alpha)(0.44 P'/P) + \alpha} \tag{25}$$

where 0.44 is an empirical adjustment factor and $\alpha = 0.2$.

N.B. The last three equations are linear relationships.

Clearance (CL) is the parameter that relates the rate of elimination to the plasma concentration.

Since

$$CL = \frac{R}{C_p^{ss}} \tag{26}$$

$$CL = \frac{V_m}{K_m + C_p^{ss}} \tag{27}$$

And since

$$\text{Apparent } t_{1/2} = \frac{0.693 \times V_d}{CL} \tag{28}$$

$$t_{1/2} = \frac{0.693 \times V_d(K_m + C_p^{ss})}{V_m} \tag{29}$$

From the above equations, it can be noted that the clearance and half-life will alter depending on the steady-state concentration. Thus V_m and K_m should be used to describe the kinetics of phenytoin and not clearance and half-life.

Selection of equations in clinical practice

In considering which equation to apply, use the algorithms shown in Figures 1.22a–c. The relevant questions are answered and the correct equation is selected from the summary of equations above.

(a) Intravenous dosing

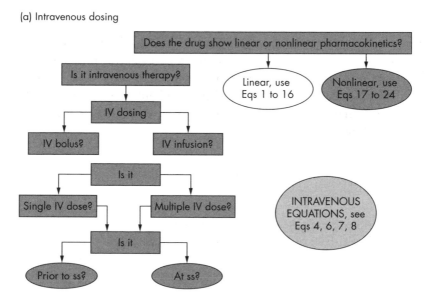

Figure 1.22 Getting the correct equation: the equation numbers link to the glossary of equations. (a) Intravenous dosing. (b) Oral dosing. (c) Loading doses and toxic level decay.

(b) Oral dosing

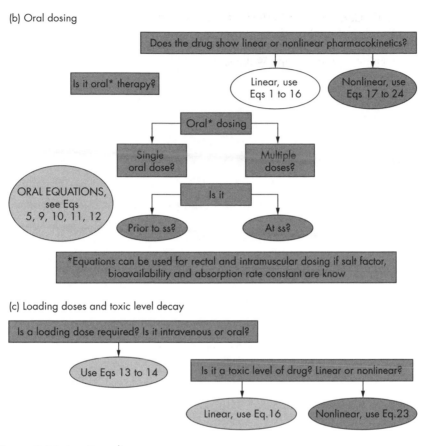

(c) Loading doses and toxic level decay

Figure 1.22 (continued).

References/Further reading

Clark, B (1986). In Clark B, Smith D A, eds. *An Introduction to Pharmacokinetics*, 2nd ed. Oxford: Blackwell Scientific.

Evans W E, Schentag J J, Jusko W J, Harrison H, eds (1992). In Evans W E, Schentag J J, eds. *Applied Pharmacokinetics: Principles of Therapeutic Drug Monitoring*, 3rd edn. Vancouver: Applied Therapeutics.

Gibaldi M, Prescott L, eds (1983). *Handbook of Clinical Pharmacokinetics*. New York: ADIS Health Science Press.

Shargel L, Wu-Pong S, Yu A B C (2005). *Applied Biopharmaceutics and Pharmacokinetics*. New York: Appleton & Lange Reviews/McGraw-Hill.

Taylor W J, Diers-Caviness M H (2003). *A Textbook of the Clinical Application of Therapeutic Drug Monitoring*. Irving, TX: Abbott Laboratories Ltd, Diagnostic Division.

White J R, Garrison M W (1994). *Basic Clinical Pharmacokinetics Handbook*. Vancouver: Applied Therapeutics.

Winter M E (2003). *Basic Clinical Pharmacokinetics*, 4th edn. Philadelphia: Lippincott Williams and Wilkins.

2

Therapeutic drug monitoring

Soraya Dhillon and Judith Cope

Aims and learning outcomes

- To explain how to establish a therapeutic drug monitoring (TDM) service.
- To describe the areas of practice that are involved in a TDM service.
- To formulate a proposal for a TDM service.

Introduction

Therapeutic drug monitoring (TDM) encompasses the measurement of serum drug levels and the application of clinical pharmacokinetics to improve patient care. The concept of clinical pharmacokinetics has been developed over the last decade. TDM is defined as the use of drug levels, pharmacokinetic principles and pharmacodynamic factors to optimise drug therapy in individual patients, and has now been developed successfully as an important area of clinical medicine.

The development of sensitive and specific methods for the determination of drug and drug metabolite concentrations in biological fluids has advanced the implementation of TDM in routine clinical practice. The interpretation of serum drug concentrations requires a knowledge of therapeutics, pharmacokinetics, drug absorption and disposition in disease states, biochemistry and pathology.

The pharmacist, through the practice of clinical pharmacy, can work with physicians and other members of the health care team to promote TDM and improve patient care. The pharmacist is well placed to identify those patients who require drug level monitoring and should aim to:

- Advise the physician on when to sample for drug level determinations
- Apply pharmacokinetic principles to help interpret the drug level

- Advise and follow up TDM requests to ensure that appropriate action is taken.

The objective of this chapter is to offer pharmacists a practical guide to establishing and developing a TDM service. Guidelines for a pharmacy-based pharmacokinetic service have been published by the Council of the Royal Pharmaceutical Society (1985). The required skills include:

- Knowledge of biopharmaceutics and pharmacokinetics and their practical application to improve quality of patient care
- Knowledge and application of therapeutics and pathology, including the effect of disease states on drug disposition
- Knowledge of the tools available in drug analysis and quality control procedures
- Written and oral communication skills
- Development, establishment and management of the service.

TDM – Which drugs and why?

For many drugs the intensity of the pharmacological effect is proportional to the drug concentration at the site of action, leading to the concept of an effective therapeutic plasma concentration range. The relationship between plasma drug concentration and clinical effect is more informative than the relationship between the drug dose and its effect. Within the optimum therapeutic concentration range, the drug exhibits maximum efficacy and minimum toxicity in the majority of patients. It is important to appreciate that the therapeutic range is a statistical concept and that for some patients the levels at which they respond or exhibit toxicity may fall outside it. Interpretation of the therapeutic range must take into account the age of the patient, the disease state for which the drug is prescribed and any reasons for altered volume of distribution or protein binding. Several examples exist where these factors will alter the therapeutic range.

The optimisation of dosage is carried out by measurement of a clinically defined endpoint for the majority of drugs (for example, antihypertensive agents and anticoagulants). Although many drugs show a wide interpatient variability in drug handling, titration of the dose can usually be made without exposing the patient to drug toxicity. Such drugs have a wide therapeutic range.

In contrast, drugs monitored routinely in serum have one or more of the following characteristics:

1. Narrow therapeutic index
2. Poor correlation between dose and effect
3. Good correlation between serum level and effect
4. Wide interpatient variation in clearance
5. A toxicity profile that is difficult to recognise clinically.

The drugs that are commonly monitored include:

1. Aminoglycosides – gentamicin, tobramycin, netilmicin, amikacin, vancomycin
2. Antiepileptic – phenytoin, carbamazepine, and occasionally phenobarbital
3. Cardioactive agents – digoxin, procainamide, lidocaine, disopyramide, flecainide
4. Others – theophylline, lithium, methotrexate, ciclosporin.

Establishing and developing a TDM service

It is important to recognise the necessity for multidisciplinary involvement in TDM. In most hospitals the laboratory services offer some form of TDM, and therefore the roles of the pharmacist and the pharmacy department depend on the extent of the individual hospital services already available. To make best use of resources, collaboration with the biochemistry and pathology department is important, especially if the assay service is based in these departments. Such an arrangement may appear to be advantageous in terms of resources, equipment, staffing and time. However, a pharmacy-based assay service offers control over the rational use of the service, and coordination of the interpretation and application of the assay results at the time they are available. The pharmacy department must examine all options before submitting its proposal.

A formal proposal for the service should be prepared, outlining the level of service offered, the cost and the benefits of the service to patients. The proposal should include:

1. Which drugs are to be measured and how the service will improve patient care
2. The rationale and justification for pharmacokinetic interpretation of the serum levels and the necessity of pharmacist involvement
3. Support from appropriate consultants or directorate managers

4. Cost (capital outlay, consumables, staff time, and transport) offset against savings made, see (5)
5. Health benefits, e.g. likely reductions in length of stay and readmission rates, optimal clinical control, rational drug usage.

Implementation of a service

The medical and administrative staff should be formally contacted and informed of the essential components of the service. TDM service documents should be designed, for example Request form and TDM information guide, and approval obtained from the medical staff concerned. It is also advisable to inform the nursing ward staff of the involvement of the pharmacy department. Request forms should be in plentiful supply on the wards and in the clinics. A guide for physicians and other health care workers should be issued to all appropriate staff indicating sampling times and therapeutic ranges. The issues that should be clear at the outset include:

*   The drugs for which the service is available
*   The days and times of assay runs
*   The latest times by which the blood sample must arrive in the laboratory for inclusion in the scheduled run
*   Request form details and how the results will be reported to the physician (verbal and/or written report)
*   The type of interpretation that pharmacy will provide and an explanation of any need for additional information.
*   'Out of hours' service to be agreed with local consultants and determined by:
    *   Clinical situations (such as overdose)
    *   Availability of staff and emergency assay techniques
    *   Other TDM services available (e.g. Poisons units)
    *   Information and pharmacokinetic advice
    *   Sample collection details – the volume of blood and the type of tube

Education and training

TDM services provided in hospital pharmacy departments should be managed and coordinated by a pharmacist supported by a deputy, each with a sound appreciation of applied pharmacokinetics. The service should be discussed among all pharmacists in the department so that it is recognised as a service commitment.

Ward pharmacists should attend seminars on each of the drugs monitored. They should always be made aware of the procedures associated with the TDM service and the importance of additional information, from drug and clinical histories to pharmacokinetic interpretation. All pharmacists must be adequately briefed on the sampling time procedure and on when and why serum levels should be monitored.

An in-service training scheme in pharmacokinetics should be implemented and each ward pharmacist given the opportunity to participate actively in the service. Regular meetings should be held to discuss TDM cases.

Interpretation of serum drug levels

The interpretation of results requires a knowledge of the patient's physical details and clinical and biochemical status. The drug history, concurrent medication, sampling details and most recent drug dosing history are also required, together with the pharmacokinetic information on the drug in question, for a valid interpretation of the serum level. Based on this information, the patient's individual pharmacokinetic parameters, i.e. the clearance (CL), volume of distribution (V_d) and elimination rate constant (k), can be estimated.

Using population pharmacokinetic data, a set of initial pharmacokinetic parameters are calculated and a level is predicted for the time the blood sample was taken. This value is compared to the assay result and the elimination rate constant is changed stepwise by iteration until the predicted level approximates the measured level. This technique can only be used if the V_d of the drug dose not vary widely. The new clearance is then calculated ($k \times V_d$) and this can be compared with the population clearance. Since population parameters are mean values, it is probable that the patient's actual parameters will lie within two standard deviations of the mean population value. If this is the case, the individualised pharmacokinetic parameters can then be used for dosage adjustments.

If the values vary widely, then the reason for this deviation should be sought; for example:

1. A check on the patient's concurrent drug therapy
2. Patient compliance
3. Drug interactions
4. Medication error

5. Change in the patient's clinical status
6. Malabsorption
7. Incorrect assay result
8. Timing of sampling
9. Site of sampling
10. Storage of sample (degradation or haemolysis).

If no explanation can be discovered for the deviation and all the factors above have been examined, then it is likely that the patient's data do differ significantly from the population mean data.

It is only then that the observed level is used to make future dosage recommendations and predictions. Any advice on alterations in dosage must be made in view of the patient's clinical condition and the assumptions and limitations of therapeutic ranges.

Free drug concentration monitoring

The measurement of concentrations of free (unbound) drug is only useful for those drugs that are highly bound to plasma proteins. Small changes in the percentage of drug bound in plasma will increase the free fraction and may alter the free concentration. In practice changes in protein binding occur in:

- Drug interactions (e.g. phenytoin and valproic acid)
- Hypoalbuminaemia (e.g. in pregnancy or liver disease)
- Elevations of plasma α_1-acid glycoprotein (e.g. following myocardial infarction)
- Saturation of binding sites (e.g. valproic acid).

For most drugs, the therapeutic range for free drug concentration in plasma is not defined and where the interpatient variation in protein binding is small may not offer advantages over the measurement of total drug concentration in plasma. Free level monitoring may be useful if protein binding interactions are suspected and can help elucidate the interaction. For example, in the presence of a protein-binding interaction, total phenytoin serum levels may be within the therapeutic range but free levels may be elevated and this may result in phenytoin toxicity.

Two methods commonly used to separate unbound and bound drug in serum are equilibrium dialysis and ultrafiltration, both of which are temperature- and time-dependent for some drugs. Ultrafiltration can be achieved by using commercially available filters (Amicon). Once separated, the free drug can be assayed by methods used to measure total plasma drug concentrations, providing they are sufficiently sensitive.

Since the salivary concentration of some drugs is equivalent to or is related to the unbound concentration, saliva may be assayed to estimate the free drug concentration, though there are many limitations to this practice.

Use of calculators and computer software packages

Pharmacokinetic interpretation of serum level data can be facilitated by using calculator or computer software packages. Early developments in TDM used existing nomograms and simple formulae to individualise dosing. These are useful providing the assumptions and disadvantages of the methods are recognised. A number of aids facilitating interpretation are now available and it is advisable to assess the individual package according to the needs of the service. A critical review of each method is beyond the scope of this chapter but, whichever software package is acquired, the user must be sure that the principles of the program, the pharmacokinetic model used, and the associated assumptions and limitations are fully understood.

A further application of pharmacokinetic modelling uses the statistical mathematics of Bayes' theorem (Sheiner and Beal, 1982). This method incorporates statistical probability and weighting for each of the drug's pharmacokinetic parameters.

For initial drug dosages the Bayesian technique may not offer any advantage over other methods. However, for drugs whose population pharmacokinetics are well defined, and when a series of serum levels in the same patient is available, the statistical weighting provided by the technique becomes increasingly relevant and advantageous. Given adequate blood level data, the Bayesian approach produces accurate and precise results.

Acknowledgement

This chapter has been reproduced with permission from UKCPA and is based on Dhillon and Cope (1995).

References/Further reading

Council of the Pharmaceutical Society (1985). *Pharm J* 234(6329): 626–627.

DHSS (1978). (Howie Report) *Code of practice for the prevention of infection in clinical laboratories and post mortem rooms*. London: HMSO.

DHSS (1986). *Revised guidelines. LAV/HTLV III, the causative agent of AIDS and related conditions*. London: DHSS.

Dhillon S, Cope J (1995). *Therapeutic Drug Monitoring (Clinical Pharmacy Practice Guide)*. UKCPA.

Evans W E, Jusko W J, Schentag J (1992). *Applied Pharmacokinetics: Principles of Therapeutic Drug Monitoring*, 3rd edn. Philadelphia: Lippincott Williams and Wilkins.

Gibaldi M, Perrier D (1982). *Pharmacokinetics*, 2nd edn. New York: Marcel Dekker.

Goodman L S, Gilman A (1985). *The Pharmacological Basis of Therapeutics*, 7th edn. London and New York: Macmillan.

Ritschel W (2004). *A Handbook of Basic Pharmacokinetics*, 6th edn. Washington DC: American Pharmaceutical Association.

Sheiner L B, Beal S L (1982). Bayesian individualisation of pharmacokinetics. Simple implementation and comparison with non-Bayesian methods. *J Pharm Sci* 71(12): 1344–1348.

Syva Ltd (1981). *Individualising Drug Therapy: Practical Applications of Drug Monitoring*. New York: Gross, Townsend, Frank Inc.

Taylor W J, Diers-Caviness M H (2003). *A Textbook of the Clinical Application of Therapeutic Drug Monitoring*. Irving, TX: Abbott Laboratories Ltd, Diagnostic Division.

Winter M E. (2004). *Basic Clinical Pharmacokinetics*, 4th edn. Philadelphia: Lippincott Williams and Wilkins.

3

Clinical pharmacokinetics in renal impairment

Caroline Ashley

Aims and learning outcomes

The aims of this chapter are to allow the reader:

- To understand the rationale for using therapeutic drug monitoring (TDM) in patients with renal impairment.
- To be able to evaluate a patient's renal function, and classify the degree of renal impairment.
- To appreciate the effects of renal dysfunction on pharmacokinetic parameters.
- To be familiar with those drugs for which TDM is important in renal impairment, and have a working knowledge of how to adjust doses according to TDM monitoring and the patient's renal function.

Rationale for therapeutic drug monitoring (TDM) in renal disease

Renal impairment has a profound effect on the disposition and handling of drugs by the body. Drugs that are excreted by the kidneys in their active form or as active metabolites are eliminated at a reduced rate. Reduced clearance causes accumulation of the drug, which can in turn lead to adverse effects. Many drugs are excreted via the renal route, and so carry an increased risk of nephrotoxicity or other end-organ damage in the presence of pre-existing renal insufficiency (Aronson, 2003). Administering the appropriate doses of drugs to patients with renal impairment is an important consideration in avoiding an increased incidence of adverse effects and ensuring optimal patient outcomes. In one survey alone, Cantu found that 44% of patients were receiving drug dosages in excess of the manufacturers' recommendation based on estimated creatinine clearance, especially with antibacterial, antiviral and antifungal agents, and cardiac glycosides (Cantu *et al.*, 1992). He also noted that a degree of renal insufficiency was present in 5% of general hospital admissions. The incidence of acute renal failure (defined as an increase in serum creatinine to 177 μmol/L or by 50% from baseline) has been quoted to be about 210 per million per year. Approximately 50% of all episodes of acute renal failure occur in patients in whom renal function was normal on admission to hospital (Armitage and Tomson, 2003).

Assessment of renal function

The kidneys remove drugs and endogenous by-products of metabolism from the body via several processes, including glomerular filtration, tubular secretion and tubular reabsorption. The rate of excretion of substances by the kidney is equal to the rate of filtration plus the rate of secretion minus the rate of reabsorption.

The assessment of glomerular filtration is fundamental to the management of drug therapy where clearance depends on renal function. Measurements of glomerular filtration rate (GFR) are based on the renal clearance of a marker in plasma, expressed as the volume of plasma completely cleared of the marker per unit time. Markers used to measure GFR include endogenous (creatinine, urea) or exogenous substances (inulin, iothalamate). The ideal marker is endogenous, freely filtered by the glomerulus, neither reabsorbed nor secreted by the renal tubule, and eliminated only by the kidney.

Inulin is considered the 'gold standard' for the estimation of GFR (Smith, 1951). Inulin is a polymer of fructose that is freely filtered by the glomerulus, and is neither reabsorbed nor secreted by the renal tubules. It is metabolically inert and is cleared only by the kidney. However, analysis of inulin is technically demanding and time-consuming. Conventional methods for estimating inulin clearance involve intravenous administration of the substance, followed by the measurement of inulin concentrations in serum and timed urine collections. Ideally, the serum levels are measured at the mid-point of the timed urine collection. The clearance is then estimated from the formula,

$$CL = \frac{C_{urine} \times V_{urine}}{C_{serum}}$$

and normalised for body surface area. Because of the technical difficulty of inulin analysis, other markers such as ^{99}Tc-DTPA, ^{51}Cr-EDTA and

^{125}I-iothalamate have been used and provide estimates of GFR that compare well with inulin.

Serum creatinine and creatinine clearance (CL$_{cr}$) remain the mainstay of the assessment of renal function, despite considerable interindividual variability in blood creatinine with muscle mass, age and sex. Although freely filtered by the glomerulus, creatinine is also secreted by the renal tubules. The extent of tubular secretion varies with renal function, which may introduce large errors in individuals with impaired renal function. A number of formulae exist to calculate CL$_{cr}$, but differences between them in accuracy and convenience mean that the two most commonly used in clinical practice are estimation of GFR using serum creatinine and urinary creatinine concentrations to calculate CL$_{cr}$.

Timed urine collection

Assuming stable renal function, CL$_{cr}$ (L/h) may be calculated using the following relationship:

$$CL_{cr} = \frac{U_{cr} \times V_{ur}}{S_{cr} \times t} \tag{3.1}$$

where U_{cr} = urine creatinine concentration (mmol/L); V_{ur} = volume of urine collected (L); S_{cr} = serum creatinine (mmol/L); and t = time interval for urine collection (h).

The traditional method of measuring urinary creatinine utilises a collection period of 24 h. However, shorter periods are as accurate and require less effort.

Cockcroft and Gault equation

The Cockcroft and Gault equation (Cockcroft and Gault, 1976) estimates creatinine clearance calculated from serum creatinine, assuming stable renal function.

$$CL_{cr} = \frac{A \times [140 - \text{Age (years)}] \times \text{Weight (kg)}}{\text{Serum creatinine } (\mu mol/L)} \tag{3.2}$$

where A = 1.23 for males, A = 1.04 for females. To normalise the calculation, it is usual practice to use ideal body weight (IBW):

IBW male = 50 + (2.3 × height in inches over 5 feet)
IBW female = 45.5 + (2.3 × height in inches over 5 feet)

There are a number of limitations to the use of the Cockcroft and Gault equation:

- It is accurate only when renal function is stable, i.e. when serum creatinine is not fluctuating by more than 40 µmol/L per day.
- It is inaccurate when serum creatinine values exceed 450 µmol/L.
- It becomes inaccurate when GFR < 20 mL/min.
- It is not valid in pregnancy.
- It is not valid in children.
- It is not valid in the very elderly.
- It is inaccurate in very wasted patients owing to decreased muscle mass.
- It is inaccurate in amputees owing to loss of muscle mass.

A number of factors may influence the production and excretion of creatinine in plasma and urine, which may artificially elevate or depress calculated CL_{cr}.

- Creatinine production depends primarily on body muscle mass, which may be radically reduced by weight loss from malnutrition, by disease, or by amputation of limbs, leading to an overestimation of CL_{cr}.
- In patients with cirrhosis, the serum creatinine concentration is typically low, and GFR is often overestimated. In such patients, direct measurement of CL_{cr} by urine collection is likely to be more accurate than equations utilising serum creatinine.
- Rapid changes in creatinine production or renal function may not be reflected in serum creatinine for several days, and steady-state conditions are necessary for accurate estimation of CL_{cr} using equations.

Renal tubular transport also has implications for the assessment of renal function. Creatinine is eliminated by both glomerular filtration and tubular secretion. The relative contribution of the latter to the overall elimination of creatinine is increased in patients with moderate to severe renal impairment. Drugs such as cimetidine and trimethoprim have been reported to increase serum creatinine levels by approximately 20% and 35%, respectively, by competitive inhibition of its secretion into the lumen of the proximal renal tubule.

Urine output

An alternative method of determining renal function is the 24-h urine collection, to estimate the amount of creatinine cleared by the kidneys during that time period. Although often inconvenient to carry out, and prone to user error, it can give an accurate measure of renal function. At the end of the collection period, a blood sample is taken to determine serum creatinine.

$$\text{GFR (mL/min)} = \frac{C_{\text{urine}} \times V_{\text{urine}}}{C_{\text{serum}}} \tag{3.3}$$

where C_{urine} = urine creatinine concentration (μmol/L); V_{urine} = volume of urine collected (mL); C_{serum} = serum creatinine concentration (μmol/L).

The volume of urine should be converted into mL/min by dividing the total volume of urine collected over 24 h by 1440 (1440 min in 24 h) before entering the value into equation (3.3). In addition, it is important to ensure that the urine concentration is entered as micromoles per litre rather than millimoles per litre as is often reported by the biochemistry laboratory.

Classification of renal failure

Once a GFR value is estimated using one of the approaches described above, the degrees of renal impairment can be classified as shown below (see Appendix 3 of the British National Formulary).

Classification	GFR (mL/min/1.73 m²)	Serum creatinine (mmol/L)
Mild	20–50	150–300
Moderate	10–20	300–700
Severe	<10	>700

Oliguria = urine output < 400 mL/day
Anuria = urine output < 50 mL/day

Altered pharmacokinetics

Reduced renal excretion is not the only change in drug disposition in patients with renal insufficiency. There are also changes in oral bioavailability, protein and tissue binding, distribution, and even hepatic metabolism. In addition, a change in drug sensitivity can alter the pharmacological or toxic response to a specific drug. Therefore, dosage adjustments should not be based solely on a decreased GFR finding.

Absorption and bioavailability

Drug absorption may be altered in patients with renal disease as a result of changes in gastric emptying time and gastric pH as well as the presence of gut oedema. Renal patients may have several causes of prolonged gastric emptying time and slow absorption of drugs from the small intestine. The most common cause is aluminium- or calcium-containing antacids used as oral phosphate binders. As well as slowing gastric motility and hence the rate of drug absorption, they can also result in decreased systemic absorption either by physically adsorbing to the drug to form insoluble complexes, or by changing gastric pH.

Other conditions that may prolong gastric emptying time include peritonitis (including CAPD peritonitis) and autonomic neuropathy in patients with diabetes mellitus, the latter representing an increasing proportion of patients on renal replacement therapy. Patients with renal dysfunction are often uraemic. The urea can be converted to ammonia by gastric urease, resulting in increased gastric pH. In addition, symptoms such as nausea, vomiting and diarrhoea are common in patients with poor renal function.

Distribution

It is generally assumed that renal impairment has little effect on the volume of distribution (V_d) of a drug. However, changes in drug distribution may arise, either from fluid retention leading to a change in the V_d of water-soluble drugs, or as a result of uraemia altering the extent of protein binding of drugs in tissue and plasma.

In patients with end-stage renal disease, the V_d of digoxin is reduced by 30–50%, postulated to be as a result of decreased tissue binding. Jusko reported that the myocardium-to-serum concentration ratio of digoxin decreased with falling creatinine clearance, so that myocardial tissue uptake of digoxin in patients with renal insufficiency may be less than in those with normal renal function (Jusko *et al.*, 1974).

The decrease in protein binding of acidic drugs observed in patients with impaired renal function may be due to several factors:

- Hypoalbuminaemia may occur in association with uraemia and in patients with nephrotic syndrome, resulting in a lower number of plasma protein molecules being available for drug binding.
- In uraemic patients, accumulated endogenous substances and/or drug metabolites can compete with acidic drugs for protein-binding

sites, displacing drugs normally bound to plasma proteins and hence increasing their free fraction, for example, of phenytoin.

• Alteration in the conformational or structural arrangement of albumin binding sites in uraemia can result in a decreased affinity of binding sites for acidic drugs.

The uraemic state induces displacement from plasma protein-binding sites, which in turn will lead to a greater free fraction of drug, and hence an increased pharmacological effect (Liponi *et al.*, 1984). However, the increased amount of unbound drug is now available for distribution and elimination. The overall effect is to reach a new steady state, where the concentration of unbound drug and the pharmacological effect in plasma are virtually the same as in individuals with normal renal function but the total plasma drug concentration is less. For example, the normal bound fraction of phenytoin is 0.9, but this is decreased to 0.8 in patients with end-stage renal disease. If the dosage is increased in patients with renal impairment to achieve the same total drug concentration as in patients with normal renal function, unbound phenytoin concentrations will be increased and toxic effects will result.

Metabolism

Although it is generally assumed that nonrenal elimination is unchanged in patients with impaired renal function, this is not necessarily true for all drugs. Various studies have documented decreases in the nonrenal clearance of several drugs, ranging from 17% (codeine) to 85% (imipenem).

The effect of renal impairment on oxidation and reduction pathways is generally minimal, except for the enhanced oxidation of phenytoin and decreased reduction of cortisol. Synthetic reactions such as sulfation (e.g. of paracetamol) and glucuronidation (e.g. of chloramphenicol) are usually normal, whereas the acetylation of isoniazid has been reported to be decreased.

Hence in patients with renal insufficiency, although the elimination of the parent compound may be unchanged, the formation of metabolites may be altered, thus affecting the overall rate and extent of excretion of the drug.

Metabolism in the kidney

The kidney, in particular the renal cortex, contains many of the same metabolic enzymes found in the liver, including cytochrome P450.

However, given that the total weight of the kidneys is considerably less than the weight of the liver, the contribution of the kidneys to total metabolic activity is probably low.

The effect of renal impairment on renal drug metabolism becomes clinically important after a few days. Metabolic activation of vitamin D (from diet or synthesised in the skin) requires hydroxylation at both the 25-position in the liver and the 1α-position in the kidney. Therefore, patients with renal impairment require administration of vitamin D in the form of 1α-hydroxycholecalciferol (alfacalcidol) or 1,25-dihydroxycholecalciferol (calcitriol) in order to increase absorption of calcium and prevent renal bone disease.

The kidney is one of the major sites of insulin degradation, which is not compensated by increased hepatic degradation. Reduced extrarenal insulin metabolism has also been reported. Hence, insulin requirements are decreased in patients with severe renal impairment, so insulin doses may need to be reduced.

The kidneys are also the major site of production of erythropoietin, the hormone that stimulates erythropoiesis. Patients with severe renal impairment develop a profound anaemia, which may now be treated with intravenous or subcutaneous injections of human recombinant erythropoietin.

Accumulation of metabolites

Patients with chronic renal insufficiency receiving long-term drug treatment may have accumulation of drug metabolites that are primarily renally excreted. Therefore, patients will be exposed to a prolonged drug effect or toxicity if a metabolite possesses pharmacological activity, particularly if a large percentage of the active metabolite is eliminated unchanged by the kidney. Osborne describes how morphine is primarily metabolised by the liver to five metabolites: morphine-3-glucuronide, morphine-6-glucuronide, normorphine, codeine and morphine-N-oxide (Osborne *et al.*, 1986). Renal excretion of unchanged morphine only accounts for 3–7% of its overall elimination, so logically morphine could be safely used in patients with renal dysfunction. However, when given standard doses of morphine, patients with severe renal impairment display classical signs of morphine toxicity, including respiratory and CNS depression and hypotension. Evidence indicates that accumulation of morphine-6-glucuronide may be the culprit. It is pharmacologically active, has been shown to cross the blood–brain barrier, and has a greater affinity for brain tissue than the parent drug morphine. Not only does it have a more potent analgesic effect, but its duration of action is also longer. It is eliminated by the kidneys, and has been shown to accumulate following administration in patients with renal impairment.

Excretion

The biological processes of glomerular filtration, active tubular excretion and passive tubular reabsorption all contribute to the net renal excretion of a drug from the body. In general, dosage adjustment in renal impairment assumes that renal disease affects all segments of the nephron, and hence these processes, equally. Therefore, regardless of whether a drug is excreted primarily by glomerular filtration or active tubular excretion, the assumption is that its renal clearance is reduced in proportion to the reduction in creatinine clearance or glomerular filtration rate. Hence, measurement or estimation of CL_{cr} is commonly used in the clinical setting for dosage adjustment in patients with renal impairment.

Approaches to drug dose alteration in renal impairment

In general, the principle is that a reduction in glomerular filtration rate (GFR) and creatinine clearance (CL_{cr}) is proportional to a concomitant reduction in drug clearance. While this is usually applicable, patients with changing renal function, differing aetiologies of renal disease and multiple co-morbid conditions may not fit published nomograms very well.

Many drugs marketed in the last 10–15 years have been studied in patients with varying degrees of renal insufficiency; hence, dosing recommendations are now provided by the manufacturer. However, these data come from studies of small numbers of patients with a narrow spectrum of renal disease, so that extrapolation to *all* renal patients is not always valid.

Maintenance dose

There are two basic methods for alteration of the maintenance dose in renal insufficiency:

1. Decrease the dose, but maintain the same dosing interval as used for patients with normal renal function.
2. Maintain the dose, but increase the dosing interval.

Both approaches may lead to an average plasma concentration similar to that observed in patients with normal renal function. However, peak or trough levels may be excessively raised or lowered. In practice, a combination of changes in both dose and dosing interval are employed according to the drug in question.

For example, aminoglycosides exert their killing action in a concentration-dependent, rather than a time-dependent, fashion and exhibit a postantibiotic effect with several organisms. Therefore, high peak concentrations are desirable, and this forms the basis of the once-daily administration of these agents. In patients with renal dysfunction, it is reasonable practice to both decrease the dose and increase the dosing interval according to measured blood drug levels (Devine, 1974). For example, a GFR > 80 mL/min requires a dose of 5.0 mg/kg every 24 h; a GFR of 30–40 mL/min warrants a dose of 2.5–3.0 mg/kg every 24 h; whereas a GFR < 10 mL/min will need a dose of only 2.0 mg/kg every 48 h (Ashley and Currie, 2003; Bennett *et al.*, 1999).

It should be remembered that both of the above dosing principles assume no change in other pharmacokinetic parameters, e.g. V_d and nonrenal clearance, which is not always the case in patients with renal impairment.

Loading dose

One other point to remember is that loading doses in renal insufficiency are in general the same as those used in patients with normal renal function. The rule of thumb that it takes approximately 4–5 half-lives to reach steady state remains true if a drug is renally excreted, but the half-life will be greatly extended, and it will thus take a longer time to reach steady state. If a therapeutic effect is required relatively quickly, then a loading dose should be given as usual. Again because of the extended half-life, it will take longer for the loading dose to be eliminated, thus allowing the amended maintenance dose to reach steady state while maintaining therapeutic efficacy.

The elderly represent a growing proportion of the total population and it is necessary to appreciate the age-associated physiological changes that occur in these patients and their effects on the disposition of drugs. Renal function is expected to decline steadily with normal ageing. The extent of the deterioration depends on the presence of concurrent disease states, for example hypertension or diabetes mellitus, which may independently impair renal function. Alterations in renal anatomy and physiology associated with ageing include decreases in renal mass, the number and size of intact nephrons, and glomerular filtration rate. Renal plasma flow has been reported to be reduced by up to 40%.

Serum creatinine varies with age, sex, diet and muscle mass. Theoretically, since elderly people have a decreased muscle mass, they should also have a lower serum creatinine compared with younger subjects, owing to the reduced production of creatinine. However, this reduction is offset by the age-related reduction in creatinine clearance, resulting in a negligible net change in observed serum creatinine. Hence an elderly person may present with a 'normal' serum creatinine, but it must be remembered that a normal GFR in an 80-year-old is considerably less than a normal GFR in a 20-year-old, and drug doses should be amended accordingly.

Creatinine clearance starts to decline by the fourth decade of life. Hence chronological age is a good and useful predictor of the elimination rate of drugs cleared primarily by glomerular filtration. The theoretical effects of a reduction in clearance in those drugs excreted unchanged via the renal route are an increase in the AUC (area under the concentration–time curve) and the elimination half-life, leading to accumulation and resulting in toxicity and an increase in the number of adverse drug events.

Drugs with a low therapeutic index and significant renal clearance, for example vancomycin, aminoglycosides, digoxin and lithium, all require plasma concentration monitoring in patients with renal impairment and in the elderly. When prescribing digoxin, it is necessary to anticipate the reduced clearance of the drug in the elderly or in renal insufficiency and adjust the dose accordingly. Thiazide diuretics are a commonly prescribed medication in the elderly population. The diuretic effect of thiazides is reduced in moderate renal insufficiency, and so therapeutic responsiveness may decline with ageing even though the serum creatinine is apparently within the normal range.

Dialysis

An increasing number of patients with end-stage renal disease receive different types of renal replacement therapy, and most of these patients are also prescribed a number of drugs. It is therefore important to know which of these drugs are removed by the various dialysis procedures, and to what extent.

Patients with chronic renal impairment who have reached end-stage renal failure are generally maintained on either intermittent haemodialysis (IHD) or peritoneal dialysis (PD). IHD involves the patient being dialysed as an outpatient for 3–5 h, three times a week. PD requires the surgical implantation of an indwelling catheter, followed by the influx and efflux of dialysis fluid 3–4 times a day. This fluid remains in the abdominal cavity for several hours at a time and utilises the peritoneum as a semipermeable dialysis membrane.

The pharmacokinetic model in IHD for renally excreted drugs is such that a maintenance drug dose produces plasma concentrations that are relatively constant between dialysis sessions. This plasma concentration represents the steady-state condition with very little fluctuation of drug concentration between doses. A rapid decline in the drug concentration corresponds to a period of haemodialysis when drug is being rapidly removed, followed by the rapid return of the plasma drug concentration to steady state, reflecting the administration of a postdialysis replacement dose.

Continuous renal replacement therapy (CRRT) is usually employed in sicker patients with cardiovascular instability who cannot tolerate the large corporeal circuit volume and fast pump speeds of IHD.

Continuous haemofiltration (CAVH/CVVH) removes solutes (waste products and drugs) by convective transport or ultrafiltration; that is, movement of fluid across a semipermeable membrane when pressure is applied to one side of that membrane. The rate of blood flow through the membrane generates the hydrostatic pressure, which forces plasma water to move across the filter, 'dragging' various solutes, including many drugs, with it.

Continuous haemodiafiltration (CAVHD/CVVHD) combines the forces of convection with diffusion (the movement of solute along a concentration gradient between plasma and dialysate) to enhance the removal of these substances. The difference in flow rate that exists, within the membrane, between the dialysis fluid (17–34 mL/min) and the blood (75–150 mL/min) allows complete equilibration to occur, resulting in the effective removal of solutes. As the solute clearance achieved by this technique is mainly a result of diffusion rather than convection, it is not necessary to generate large volumes of ultrafiltrate and consequently the volume of replacement fluid required, compared with haemofiltration, is reduced.

When evaluating drug removal by dialysis, the pharmacokinetic and pharmacodynamic properties of the drug, as well as the type of dialysing membrane and flow settings all need to be considered.

Drug characteristics

- Conventional dialysis readily removes free drug molecules with a molecular weight less than 500 daltons (Da). Drugs with a molecular weight between 500 and 2000 Da are inadequately removed, and drugs with a weight greater than 2000 Da (e.g. vancomycin, MW = 3300 Da) are not removed at all. Note that high-flux dialysis filters, and those used for CAVH/CAVHD, have the capacity to dialyse larger molecules and so will remove vancomycin to an extent.
- Drugs that are water-soluble are more readily removed by dialysis, while lipid-soluble drugs are difficult to remove.
- Drugs with a large V_d (i.e. lipid-soluble drugs or those with a high degree of tissue binding) are less concentrated in the blood and therefore tend not to be removed by haemodialysis. Accordingly, drugs with a small V_d (<1 L/kg) are more easily dialysed, while those with a large V_d (>2 L/kg) are poorly dialysed.
- Drugs with a low degree of protein binding are more readily dialysed, as more unbound drug is available to cross the dialysis membrane.
- Drugs with a short half-life tend to be more readily removed by dialysis.
- Drugs that are normally cleared by the kidneys in patients with normal renal function have characteristics favouring their adequate removal by haemodialysis.

Dialyser characteristics

- Given the same dialyser material, the greater the surface area of the dialyser membrane, the greater is the amount of drug removed.
- Increasing the blood flow rate presents a larger amount of drug to the dialyser membrane for removal.
- Increasing the dialysate flow rate will keep the dialysate drug concentration at a minimum and thus maintain the concentration gradient across the membrane.

When determining the amount of drug removed by dialysis, or the post-dialysis concentration, it is also necessary to consider the redistribution phenomenon, i.e. a rebound in serum drug concentration that occurs after dialysis. This occurs if the rate of removal of a drug from the blood during dialysis is greater than the rate of movement of the drug from tissue stores back to the blood. In this situation, the use of a predialysis and postdialysis serum concentration may overestimate the ability of the dialysis process to remove drugs.

Table 3.1 Typical clearance values achieved by commonly used renal replacement techniques

Renal replacement technique[a]	Mode of action	Type of renal failure used to treat	Typical clearance (mL/min)
CAPD	Dialysis and ultrafiltration	Chronic	5–8
Intermittent HD	Dialysis and ultrafiltration	Chronic	150–200
CAVH	Ultrafiltration only	Acute	10–20
CVVH	Ultrafiltration only	Acute	Up to 50
CAVHD or CVVHD	Dialysis and ultrafiltration	Acute	20–25

[a] Refer to list of abbreviations.

Although a large amount of literature is available on drug clearance in patients receiving renal replacement therapy, it should be used with caution. There are a multitude of renal replacement therapies available, which have a variety of different clearance characteristics. The usual measure of renal replacement therapy function – urea clearance – is similar to creatinine clearance. It can be added to the patient's own inherent renal function (usually zero owing to anuria) to calculate dosages of dialysable drugs. Modern dialysis systems have the approximate clearances shown in Table 3.1.

Loading doses of drugs

Drugs that are principally cleared by the kidneys, such as gentamicin or digoxin, will accumulate if given in conventional doses to patients with renal failure; either a reduced dose or an increased dosing interval should be employed. However, as the latter will delay the time taken for the drug to achieve the desired plasma steady-state concentration (usually 4.5 × the drug's elimination half-life), an initial loading dose may need to be given for certain drugs. The loading dose can be calculated from a knowledge of the drug's apparent volume of distribution (V_d), the patient's weight and the plasma level desired (C_p) using the equation (Winter, 2003):

$$\text{Loading dose (mg)} = [V_d \ (\text{L/kg}) \times \text{weight (kg)}] \times C_p \ (\text{mg/L})$$

(3.4)

Although the reported changes in the volume of distribution of some drugs in critically ill patients limits the accuracy of this approach (Bodenham *et al.*, 1988), it is generally recommended that standard loading doses should be administered to patients receiving continuous renal replacement. The validity of doses calculated using equation (3.4) depends on a close relationship existing between the plasma concentration measured and the therapeutic efficacy of the drug.

Administration of maintenance doses in renal replacement therapy

A number of different approaches can be used to estimate the maintenance dose that should be administered to patients receiving either continuous haemofiltration or haemodialysis. The simplest method is to choose a dose based on an estimate of the creatinine clearance (CL_{cr}) achieved by the extracorporeal system used. For haemofiltration systems, the volume of ultrafiltrate (UFR) collected each hour can be used to represent the CL_{cr}; for example, a UFR volume of 1800 mL/h = CL_{cr} of 30 mL/min (assuming for creatinine a sieving coefficient, S, of 1). When the UFR volume is greater than 15 mL/min, the dose selected should reflect that administered to patients with moderate renal impairment; when the UFR is less than 15 mL/min, the dose used should follow that recommended for patients with severe renal impairment. Continuous haemodiafiltration systems, employing a dialysis flow rate of 1–2 litres per hour, normally achieve a CL_{cr} of between 20 and 30 mL/min, which can be used to select a dose by following guidelines given for patients with moderate renal impairment.

A second approach is to use the sieving coefficient (S) value of a drug (or the fraction of non-protein-bound drug if S is unknown) to determine the extracorporeal clearance. The sieving coefficient of a drug is the proportion that will pass through the haemofiltration membrane during a period of pure ultrafiltration and is largely dependent on its physiochemical properties. The sieving coefficient is analogous to the partition coefficient of a compound and provides useful data on the likely removal of a drug by continuous haemodiafiltration. This relationship can be expressed mathematically as

$$S = \frac{C_{UFR}}{C_{arterial}} \qquad (3.5)$$

where S = sieving coefficient; C_{UFR} = concentration of drug in ultra-filtrate; and $C_{arterial}$ = concentration of drug in the arterial circulation (i.e. prefilter concentration of drug).

A drug that freely passes through the membrane during ultrafiltration alone will have a sieving coefficient of 1; whereas a drug that is not removed at all by the process will have an S value of 0. Sieving coefficient values are unique to the filter system used to generate the data. However, for practical purposes, S values are commonly used regardless of the system used to generate the results. The system variables most likely to influence clearance data are the blood flow to the filter, the type of membrane used, the ultrafiltration rate and, in continuous haemo-diafiltration, the dialysis fluid flow rate.

The extracorporeal clearance of a drug during continuous haemo-filtration, CL_{hf}, can then be calculated from a knowledge of the sieving coefficient and the ultrafiltration volume collected over a known period of time:

$$CL_{hf} = S \times UFR \text{ (L/h)} \qquad (3.6)$$

where UFR is the average ultrafiltration rate recorded.

Sieving coefficients calculated during haemodialysis represent the proportion of a drug removed from the circulation by the combined forces of dialysis and ultrafiltration. This will be influenced by the dialysate flow rate and the type of membrane.

Conclusion

Renal impairment will have marked effects on the pharmacokinetic and pharmacodynamic properties of renally excreted drugs. Various factors have to be taken into account when prescribing for such patients, in order to maximise therapeutic efficacy but at the same time minimise both nephrotoxicity and other end-organ damage. Specialist advice should be sought if appropriate.

Clinical case studies

Cases studies 3.1 and 3.2 present some clinical case examples.

● **CASE STUDY 3.1**

Mrs R.M., aged 86 years (weight 51 kg, height 155 cm (5 ft 1 in.) is admitted with presenting complaints of recent unexplained falls, no appetite, nausea, abdominal pain and diarrhoea, constant fatigue and confusion. She has a previous medical history of atrial fibrillation and drugs on admission were digoxin 250 μg o.d. and paracetamol 1 g q.d.s. p.r.n.

Serum biochemistry:

Urea	9.8 mmol/L (range 3.0–6.5)
Creatinine	96 μmol/L (range 60–100)
Potassium	4.4 mmol/L (range 3.5–5.0)
Sodium	147 mmol/L (range 135–145)
Calcium	2.51 mmol/L (range 2.1–2.6)
Phosphate	0.99 mmol/L (range 0.87–1.45)
Albumin	28 g/L (range 35–50)
Digoxin level	3.67 ng/mL (range 0.8–2.0 ng/mL)

Is the current digoxin therapy satisfactory?
Calculate creatinine clearance using the Cockcroft and Gault equation:

$$CL_{cr} = \frac{[1.04(140 - 86) \times 51]}{96}$$
$$= 29.8 \, mL/min$$

Calculate Mrs R.M.'s digoxin clearance from population data, without heart failure:

$$\begin{aligned} CL_{dig} &= 0.06 \times CL_{cr} + 0.05 \times IBW \\ &= 0.06 \times 29.8 + 0.05 \times 47.8 \\ &= 1.786 + 2.39 \\ &= 4.178 \, L/h \end{aligned}$$

Calculate Mrs R.M.'s predicted steady-state concentration from population data:

$$\begin{aligned} C_p^{ss} &= \frac{S \times F \times D}{CL \times \tau} \\ &= \frac{[1 \times 0.63 \times 250]}{[4.178 \times 24]} \\ &= 1.57 \, ng/mL \end{aligned}$$

→

> **CASE STUDY 3.1** (continued)

Calculate Mrs R.M.'s observed digoxin clearance based on measured serum digoxin levels:

$$CL_{obs} = \frac{S \times F \times D}{C_p^{ss} \times \tau}$$

$$= \frac{[0.63 \times 1 \times 250]}{[3.67 \times 24]}$$

$$= \frac{157.5}{88.08}$$

$$= 1.788 \, L/h$$

It can be seen that Mrs R.M. is clearing her digoxin dose at approximately one-quarter the rate of someone with normal renal function.

Calculate the average volume of distribution for digoxin:

$$V_d = 7.3 \, L/kg$$

$$= 7.3 \times 51$$

$$= 372.3 \, L$$

Calculate Mrs R.M.'s elimination rate constant based on observed data:

$$k = \frac{CL}{V_d}$$

$$= \frac{1.788}{372.3}$$

$$= 0.0048 \, h^{-1}$$

Using this, we can calculate how long it will be before Mrs R.M.'s serum digoxin level will once more be within the normal range:

$$\text{Time to decay} = \frac{\ln C_{p1} - \ln C_{p2}}{k_{el}}$$

$$= \frac{\ln(3.67/1.5)}{0.0048}$$

$$= 186 \, h$$

$$= \sim 8 \, \text{days}$$

$\rightarrow$

CASE STUDY 3.1 (continued)

Now calculate a new maintenance dose for Mrs R.M. based on her observed clearance data:

$$\text{Maintenance dose} = \frac{CL \times C_{p\,ave}^{ss} \times \tau}{S \times F}$$
$$= \frac{1.788 \times 1.5 \times 24}{1 \times 0.63}$$
$$= 102.17 \, \mu g$$

Hence the advice for Mrs R.M. would be to withhold any further digoxin doses for 8 days, then re-check her serum digoxin level to ensure that she is now within the therapeutic range, then recommence therapy at a maintenance dose of 125 µg daily, and re-check levels once steady state has again been reached. Unless Mrs R.M. is extremely symptomatic or showing signs of ECG changes, it is unlikely that Digibind therapy will be necessary in this instance.

CASE STUDY 3.2

Mrs A.B., aged 66 years, was admitted recently under the plastic surgery team for the excision of a malignant melanoma. She made an uneventful recovery, and was discharged, to return to the unit for dressing changes and assessment. Her serum creatinine on discharge was 93 µmol/L. On her return one week later, the wound was red and inflamed, the patient was pyrexial with a temperature of 38.6°C, and wound swabs were positive for Acinetobacter baumannii.

Mrs A.B. is admitted for the treatment of her wound infection. Blood cultures, full blood count and urea and electrolytes are also measured. Mrs A.B.'s weight is 82 kg and her height is 167.6 cm (5 ft 6 in.).

Mrs A.B. is given 400 mg gentamicin in the clinic, then admitted to the ward, where she is prescribed gentamicin 650 mg IV once daily. The ward staff do not realise that the first dose of gentamicin has already been administered in clinic, and so administer the second dose.

→

CASE STUDY 3.2 (continued)

Just after the gentamicin is given, her serum creatinine is reported by the laboratory as 171 μmol/L.

What would you advise?
From the Cockcroft and Gault equation:

$$CL_{cr} = \frac{1.04(140 - Age) \times Weight}{Serum\ creatinine}$$

$$= \frac{1.04(140 - 66) \times 59.3\ (IBW)}{171}$$

$$= 26.7\ mL/min$$

There are two points to be noted here:

- Before prescribing or administering potentially toxic drugs that are renally cleared, always re-check the patient's renal function. Even though Mrs A.B.'s was normal a week ago, she is now clearly septic, which can cause marked deterioration of renal function, as seems to have occurred in Mrs A.B.'s case.
- Gentamicin doses should always be calculated according to the patient's ideal body weight. The first dose Mrs A.B. was given was prescribed in this way, at 7 mg/kg, but the second dose was calculated according to her actual body weight. This compounded the overdose problem, leading to even further toxicity.

Given Mrs A.B.'s actual renal function, she should have been prescribed a reduced dose, for example 3.0–3.5 mg/kg, and levels monitored until her trough level was <1.5 mg/L.

Over the next few days, her serum creatinine rose dramatically:

Day	Serum creatinine (μmol/L)	Serum gentamicin level (mg/L)
1	171	–
2	370	21.7
3	529	16.0
4	736	13.8

→

Calculating Mrs A.B.'s parameters:
Elimination rate constant:

$$k = \frac{\ln C_{p1} - \ln C_{p2}}{t}$$
$$= \frac{\ln(21.7/16.0)}{24}$$
$$= \frac{0.3047}{24}$$
$$= 0.0127 \, h^{-1}$$

where t = time (h) between the two levels being taken.

Half-life:

$$t_{1/2} = \frac{0.693}{0.0127} = 54.6 \, h$$

If the measured plasma level of 21.7 mg/L was taken 14 h after the 650 mg dose of gentamicin was administered, we can extrapolate back to calculate the original peak concentration:

$$C_p^0 = \frac{C_p}{\exp(-kt)}$$
$$= \frac{21.7}{0.8371}$$
$$= 25.92 \, mg/L$$

Volume of distribution:

$$V_d = \frac{D}{C_{p \, peak} - C_{p \, min}}$$
$$= \frac{400 + 650}{25.92 - 16.0}$$
$$= \frac{1050}{105.8}$$
$$= 105.8 \, L$$

$\rightarrow$

> **◗ CASE STUDY 3.2** (continued)
>
>
> Work out how long it will take Mrs A.B. to excrete the cumulative doses of gentamicin and achieve a trough level of 1.5mg/L:
>
> $$C^{ss}_{p\,min} = C^{ss}_{p\,max} \times \exp(-k\tau)$$
>
> Therefore,
>
> $$C^{ss}_{p\,min}/C^{ss}_{p\,max} = \exp(-k\tau) = 0.05787$$
> $$-k\tau = -2.8496$$
> $$\tau = 224\,h$$
>
> i.e. it will take Mrs A.B. over 9 days to excrete the gentamicin. The persistence of high plasma concentrations will place her at increased risk of developing ototoxicity and further nephrotoxicity, so it may be prudent to given Mrs A.B. haemodialysis to remove the majority of the drug. As well as minimising the risk of further toxicity, this will also improve the chances of her regaining renal function.

In practice, in patients with moderate to severe renal impairment, it is usual to administer a reduced dose (moderate renal impairment = 3.0–5.0 mg/kg/day and severe renal impairment = 2.0–3.0 mg/kg/day), and withhold further doses until it has been ascertained that the patient's trough level is <1.5–2.0 mg/L. This approach is especially useful where the patient has changing renal function, so that any pharmacokinetic parameters calculated are liable to alter, making dosage adjustment difficult.

If a patient is on dialysis, gentamicin elimination will be irregular, occurring at much higher rates during the dialysis, and so maintenance dose calculations cannot be used. One commonly used approach is to administer aminoglycosides only after each dialysis session. The dose used is the amount of drug lost during the interdialytic as well as intradialytic period, and is commonly 2.0 mg/kg.

CASE STUDY 3.3

Mrs H.K. is a 52-year-old lady in end-stage renal failure (ESRF), who is on inter-mittent haemodialysis three times a week. She has been admitted for refashioning of her arterio-venous fistula used for dialysis access.

PMH: *ESRF for last 12 years, secondary to adult polycystic kidney disease. Epilepsy (grand mal fits) since childhood.*

Her current antiepileptic medication is phenytoin 200 mg once daily.

While Mrs H.K. is an inpatient, her steady-state plasma phenytoin level is measured and reported to be 7.0 mg/L. The doctor wants to increase the dose to 300 mg once daily.

What would you advise?

Weight	38.5 kg
Height	155 cm
Serum albumin	29 g/L
Serum sodium	136 mmol/L
Serum potassium	4.7 mmol/L
Serum calcium	2.26 mmol/L
Serum magnesium	0.97 mmol/L
Serum phosphate	1.89 mmol/L
Serum urea	18.2 mmol/L
Serum creatinine	463 μmol/L

It is imperative that plasma phenytoin concentrations are critically evaluated in patients with end-stage renal disease for two reasons:

- Plasma protein binding of drugs is altered in uraemic individuals, where the increased plasma urea levels leads to plasma proteins having a decreased binding affinity for drugs, especially acidic drugs.
- Patients with end-stage renal disease often have a low serum albumin.

In patients with normal renal function, approximately 90% of the measured plasma phenytoin concentration is bound to albumin and 10% is free. In uraemic, hypoalbuminaemic patients, with very poor renal function, the free fraction increases to a range of 20–35%, as reported by Liponi (Liponi *et al.*, 1984). In patients with renal failure who have a normal serum albumin, the free fraction is approximately 20%.

Since the free fraction (α) for phenytoin is increased in uraemic individuals, lower plasma concentrations will produce pharmacological effects that are equivalent to those produced by higher levels in normal individuals. This can be shown in Mrs H.K. by adjusting her measured plasma phenytoin level for both uraemia and hypoalbuminaemia. Ideal body weight = 47.8 kg, therefore

→

CASE STUDY 3.3 (continued)

use the patient's actual body weight in all calculations. Adjusting the patient's phenytoin level just for hypoalbuminaemia, but not for uraemia, we see that:

$$C_{p\,adjusted} = \frac{C_p^*}{(1 - \alpha)[P'/P] + \alpha}$$

$$= \frac{C_p^*}{(1 - 0.1)[\text{Patient's albumin}/(44\,g/L)] + 0.1}$$

$$= \frac{7}{0.9 \times [29/44] + 0.1}$$

$$= \frac{7}{0.9 \times 0.66 + 0.1}$$

$$= 10.09\,mg/L$$

However, adjusting the patient's phenytoin level for both hypoalbuminaemia and uraemia, we see that:

$$C_{p\,adjusted} = \frac{C_p^*}{(0.48)(1 - \alpha)[P'/P] + \alpha}$$

$$= \frac{C_p^*}{(0.48)(1 - 0.1)[\text{Patient's albumin}/(44\,g/L)] + 0.1}$$

$$= \frac{7}{0.48 \times 0.9 \times [29/44] + 0.1}$$

$$= \frac{7}{0.48 \times 0.9 \times [0.66] + 0.1}$$

$$= 18.18\,mg/L$$

where 0.48 represents the decreased affinity for phenytoin binding to serum albumin. It was validated in patients with end stage renal disease on haemodialysis.

Therefore, Mrs H.K.'s measured plasma phenytoin concentration of 7 mg/L is comparable to a concentration of approximately 18 mg/L in a patient with normal renal function and normal serum albumin. The usually accepted therapeutic range for phenytoin in nonuraemic patients is 10–20 mg/L, so Mrs H.K.'s adjusted level corresponds to the upper end of this range. Since her seizure disorder is well controlled, and she is not displaying any overt signs of phenytoin toxicity, then there need be no adjustment to her current phenytoin dose.

The amount of phenytoin removed by dialysis is negligible, and dialysis does not change the protein binding characteristics of the drug. Therefore, doses do not need to be adjusted merely because the patient is on dialysis. Changes in plasma protein binding occur within a few days following the onset of acute renal failure. Interestingly, there is some evidence that following successful renal transplantation, the plasma protein binding of phenytoin increases rapidly over the first 2–4 postoperative days, and is almost normal at 2 weeks.

References/Further reading

Armitage A J, Tomson C (2003). Acute renal failure. *Medicine* 31(6): 43–48.

Aronson J K (2003). Drugs and renal insufficiency. *Medicine* 31(7): 103–109.

Ashley C A, Currie A (2003). *Renal Drug Handbook*, 2nd edn. Abingdon: Radcliffe Medical Press.

Bennett W M, Aronoff G R, Berns J S *et al.* (1999). *Drug Prescribing in Renal Failure. Dosing Guidelines for Adults*, 4th edn. Philadelphia: American College of Physicians.

Bodenham A, Shelly M P, Park G R (1988). The altered pharmacokinetics and pharmacodynamics of drugs commonly used in critically ill patients. *Clin Pharmacokinet* 14: 347–373.

Cantu T G, Ellerbeck E D, Yun S W (1992). Drug prescribing for patients with changing renal function. *Am J Hosp Pharm* 49: 2944–2948.

Cockcroft D W, Gault M H (1976). Prediction of creatinine clearance from serum creatinine. *Nephron* 16: 31–41.

Devine B J (1974). Gentamicin therapy. *Drug Intell Clin Pharm* 7: 650–655.

Gault M H, Longerich L L, Harnett J D, Wesolowski C (1992). Predicting glomerular function from adjusted serum creatinine. *Nephron* 62: 249–256.

Jusko W J, Szefler S J, Goldfarb A L (1974). Pharmacokinetic design of digoxin dosage regimens in relation to renal function. *J Clin Pharmacol* 14: 525–535.

Liponi D L, Winter M E, Tozer T N *et al.* (1984). Renal function and therapeutic concentrations of phenytoin. *Neurology* 34: 395.

Osborne R, Joel S P, Slevin M L (1986). Morphine intoxication in renal insufficiency: the role of morphine-6-glucuronide. *BMJ* 292: 1548–1549.

Smith H W, ed. (1951). *The Kidney: Structure and Function in Health and Disease*. New York: Oxford University Press, 231–238.

Winter M E (2003). *Basic Clinical Pharmacokinetics*, 4th edn. Philadelphia: Lippincott Williams and Wilkins.

4

The effect of liver dysfunction on pharmacokinetics

Caron Weeks and Mark Tomlin

Aims and learning outcomes

To describe the effect of liver dysfunction on drug handling:

- Understanding the rationale for therapeutic drug monitoring.
- Understanding the principles involved.
- Understanding the tools that can be used to assess the drug-metabolising function of liver.
- Understanding clinical practice.
- Illustrating action with case studies.

Introduction

The liver plays a central role in the absorption and disposition kinetics of most drugs (Verbeeck and Horsman, 1998). Parameters such as liver blood flow, binding to plasma proteins and biliary excretion, all of which can potentially influence drug pharmacokinetics, depend upon the normal functioning of the liver. Age, genetics and drug interactions can produce huge variability in liver enzyme function. Co-morbidities such as cardiac function, thyroid status, diabetes, alcohol intake and pregnancy are also important.

Liver disease can be subdivided into cholestasis, cirrhosis, hepatitis, hepatoma and porphyria, and these appear to differ in their effects on drug clearance. It is vital to understand the mechanism of drug clearance by the liver and to combine this with knowledge of how the different types of liver dysfunction affect enzyme systems.

Most of the information available on the altered handling of drugs has come from patients with cirrhosis. Cirrhosis is a diffuse process characterised by fibrosis and a conversion of normal architecture into structurally abnormal nodules (Verbeeck and Horsman, 1998). These modifications are associated with and/or responsible for a reduction in liver blood supply, the presence of intra- and extrahepatic portosystemic shunting, a capillarisation of the sinusoids, a reduction in the number and in the activity of the hepatocytes, and impairment of the production of albumin. Such progression will lead to the development of clinical manifestations such as varices, oedema, ascites, severe impairment of parenchymal function and hepatic encephalopathy. This may contribute to alterations in the pharmacokinetic behaviour of many drugs. Impaired secretion of bile acids, bilirubin and other organic anions is also observed in cirrhosis, mainly when its aetiology is linked to lesions of the extrahepatic biliary tract. Besides these phenomena, cirrhosis may also exert a major influence on other organs such as the intestines, the lungs and the kidneys (the hepatorenal syndrome).

There are no clear markers of liver dysfunction, unlike renal dysfunction where urine output and creatinine clearance are reliable predictors of renal clearance. Standard liver function tests such as rises in alkaline phosphatase and alanine aminotransferase are only crude markers of liver performance and have not proved to be useful in characterising liver function in relation to drug pharmacokinetics. These tests show that liver damage has occurred and some liver function has been lost, but do not show what level of liver function remains. Thus, despite many drugs being eliminated by liver biotransformation, there is a lack of data about how liver dysfunction will alter drug clearance (Curry, 1974).

It is therefore not surprising that the effect of liver dysfunction on drug clearance is often a descriptive, quantitative prediction and calculations are rare. Model drugs can be used to describe the effect of liver function on drug metabolism. These drug models are, however, research tools and not part of common clinical practice.

The effect of liver dysfunction on drug handling is often unpredictable as some changes are due to the way the body deals with the drug (pharmacokinetics) and some due to the way the drug affects the body (pharmacodynamics) (Curry, 1974). However, those drugs most affected by changes in liver dysfunction are those that are normally extensively cleared by the liver, those with a high liver extraction ratio, those highly bound to plasma proteins, or those with narrow therapeutic ranges or with saturable kinetics.

An understanding of the relationship between liver function and drug handling is important to ensure that dosing is adjusted to avoid drug toxicity.

Rationale for therapeutic drug monitoring (TDM)

Patients show a wide variation in both the extent of liver biotransformation and the range of metabolic pathways used to eliminate drugs. This variation is the product of the genetics of the individual as well as the influence of environmental exposure to enzyme inducers, inhibitors and interactions. This variation in metabolism of xenobiotics is not represented by normal clinical signs or biochemical tests. It manifests itself only when the patient is exposed to the medication. In addition, liver dysfunction can reveal otherwise hidden drug toxicities such as glutathione depletion with paracetamol.

The liver is a large organ, but it can lose a significant percentage of its mass while retaining its metabolic function. Biochemical indicators show only cell damage, and not the extent of mass remaining. They provide only limited information about the ability of the liver to metabolise foreign compounds such as drugs.

There is no reliable way of predicting which drugs will be metabolised. Drugs of similar structures or pharmacology still show variation in their elimination route. Beta-blockers have an enormous variation in the extent of hepatic or renal elimination. Propranolol is hepatically eliminated, atenolol is renally eliminated, and metoprolol has both hepatic and renal elimination. The extent of liver metabolism may also vary. Benzodiazepines such as diazepam and chlordiazepoxide undergo oxidative metabolism, whereas lorazepam and oxazepam undergo direct glucuronidation. Liver dysfunction will affect these therapeutic groups to different degrees.

Old age does not show a linear deterioration in metabolic function. In premature and full-term neonates, enzymes may be poorly developed generally and specific metabolic pathways may be absent. Enzyme maturation is complete by 6–8 months of age. The hepatic metabolic capacity continues to increase to a peak, at 16 years of age, and reduces thereafter. Therefore a child, who has a relatively large liver, may require a larger mg/kg dose than an adult (Curry, 1974). This is illustrated by theophylline dosing in neonate, child and adult.

The concentration of albumin in the blood normally reflects the liver synthetic rate. However, it also undergoes rapid falls as the individual becomes unwell (owing to changes in vascular permeability). In liver dysfunction, acute changes may reduce the albumin concentration by both mechanisms. Albumin itself is therefore an unreliable marker of liver dysfunction.

At the same time, highly bound drugs will have their free fraction altered and thus (for low-extraction drugs) their clinical effect and rate of clearance will change. Normally, as the free fraction increases, the liver clearance increases, but in liver dysfunction blood levels may rise significantly because the liver lacks the capacity to metabolise more drug.

Pharmacokinetic parameters

Drug delivery rate

An important variable of drug elimination is the rate of drug delivery to the organ of elimination. Global perfusion is determined by cardiac output. Cardiac output is important for drugs cleared by the liver (or kidneys).

Portal hypertension may divert blood away from the liver. Within the liver, disease may decrease overall liver blood flow as well as directing the blood flow to different parts (shunting). The most highly perfused areas may not be those with most functional enzymes.

Elimination

The enzyme capacity within hepatocytes may change as well as the number of hepatocytes, producing significant changes in enzyme functional capacity. To examine the effect of liver disease on drug elimination it is usual to look at changes in half-life. This is done simply for ease of comprehension, because elimination rate constants (k) are so cumbersome. The elimination rate constant can be determined graphically as the slope of a plot of log concentration against time. In liver failure both the volume of distribution (V_d) and total clearance (CL) may change. In liver failure the volume of distribution of tolbutamide changes, clearance of antipyrine changes, and both V_d and CL change for propranolol, lidocaine and diazepam.

Clearance

The basic premise of pharmacokinetic calculations is that the average steady-state concentration (C_p^{ss}) is determined by the drug delivery rate (R = input rate) and the output or clearance rate (CL):

$$C_p^{ss} = \frac{R}{CL}$$

where $R = SFD/\tau$; F = fraction absorbed; S = salt factor; D = dose; and τ = dosing interval.

The amount of drug assayed from a blood sample is the total of bound and unbound drug. This is important because it is the unbound drug that is pharmacologically active. For drugs of high extraction ratio, both bound and free drug are metabolised (see later), but for low-extraction drugs only unbound drug is available for clearance. With low extraction, it is assumed that more free drug will increase the rate of removal. However, in organ dysfunction this may not be true.

Clearance can be further broken down into clearance by different organs. The sum of the clearances by all organs is the total body clearance:

$$CL_{total} = CL_{renal} + CL_{liver} + CL_{lungs} + CL_{gut}, \text{ etc.}$$

Clearance is a complex mix of perfusion and eliminating capacity of the different organs. The brain is highly perfused but rarely eliminates drugs; equally the skin or gastrointestinal tract may be metabolically active but poorly perfused.

Extraction ratio

One of the dominant factors in liver kinetics is the extraction ratio (E):

$$CL = Q_b \times E$$

where Q_b = blood flow to the organ. The extraction ratio varies between 0 and 1 and describes the amount of drug that is eliminated from the blood compared to the total quantity in the blood. Total body elimination would view the whole body as one eliminating organ. More usually there is extraction by liver, lung or kidneys.

High extraction

When the extraction ratio becomes close to 1, the liver is able to eliminate all the drug in the blood passing through it. This means that liver clearance is dependent only on blood flow through the liver (Zimmerman, 1999). Therefore, drugs with high extraction by the liver are very sensitive to altered liver blood flow (Verbeeck and Horsman, 1998). Examples of drugs with high liver extraction ratios include clomethiazole, verapamil, morphine, propranolol and lidocaine.

Drugs with a high extraction ratio usually undergo significant first-pass metabolism. It is worth noting that for any drug that undergoes significant first-pass metabolism the oral and parenteral doses are different, because parenteral preparations will not be subject to first-pass metabolism.

Being bound to plasma proteins does not protect drugs with high extraction. Liver elimination is a more powerful force than that causing association between drug and plasma protein. The liver is therefore able to eliminate drug by pulling it off the plasma proteins. Effectively, both bound and free drug can be metabolised by the liver, so that changes in protein binding do not directly affect clearance.

Drugs with high extraction ratio, being dependent on liver perfusion, will also show sensitivity to changes in cardiac dysfunction. Disease states, including liver diseases, associated with alterations in liver blood flow will have a significant impact on the elimination kinetics of these drugs. Liver blood flow is altered in cirrhosis and this may also decrease first-pass metabolism. In cirrhosis the altered bioavailability of highly extracted drugs is increased in patients with a collateral circulation.

Low extraction

When the extraction ratio tends towards zero, the liver finds it difficult to eliminate the drug in the blood as it passes through. Blood flow therefore becomes less important unless the blood flow is severely restricted, leading to hepatic damage. The factors that vary the ability to remove the drug (extraction) from the blood become the rate-limiting steps that alter clearance. Drugs with low extraction ratios include theophylline, phenytoin, tolbutamide, diazepam and warfarin.

The hepatic clearance of poorly extracted drugs is mainly influenced by changes in plasma protein binding and the intrinsic hepatic clearance of the unbound drug. Plasma protein binding changes are important because bound drug may be unavailable for liver extraction. The forces drawing the drug to bind to the liver enzymes are less powerful than the forces holding the drug to the plasma proteins. Elimination by the liver is determined by the functionality of the enzymes within it.

Clearance of low-extraction drugs is said to be enzyme capacity-limited, and hepatocellular damage results in impaired clearance. Therefore, this category can be further subdivided into binding-sensitive (highly protein bound in plasma (>90%); e.g. phenytoin, warfarin) and binding-insensitive drugs (not highly protein bound, so that changes in binding do not give rise to significant changes in free levels; e.g. aminophylline).

Theophylline has a low extraction ratio and the half-life increases from 7 to 26 h in cirrhosis, owing to decreased metabolic liver activity (Widdop, 1985). Diazepam and phenytoin also have a low extraction ratio: half-life in uraemic patients (urea displacement) is much shorter than in healthy volunteers (Gibaldi, 1984).

The three variables involved in liver clearance are CL_{int}, the intrinsic clearance of the liver enzymes; Q_b, the drug delivery rate = liver blood flow; f_u, the proportion of unbound drug. From these:

$$CL_{liver} = \frac{Q_b \times f_u \times CL_{int}}{Q_b + f_u \times CL_{int}}$$

This equation is important for drugs of low extraction ratio but simplifies for drugs of high extraction ratio.

Protein binding

Chronic liver disease (e.g. cirrhosis) is usually accompanied by reduced synthesis of albumin, leading to hypoalbuminaemia and reduced drug binding to plasma proteins. The protein binding affinity may be altered in liver disease as a result of the accumulation of bilirubin and endogenous products of metabolism. These compounds, including urea, may displace drugs from their binding sites, either by direct competition or by altering the nature of the binding site.

Reduced liver synthesis may produce hypoalbuminaemia and reduced levels of alpha-acid glycoprotein (α_1-GP). This may be responsible for decreased protein binding, increasing the free fraction of some highly bound drugs by as much as 50–100%. Albumin binds acidic and neutral drugs, whereas α_1-GP binds basic drugs. However, the concentration of both of these proteins will change with sepsis and stress, so that during an acute phase of illness protein binding may change independently of liver synthesis rates. Lidocaine undergoes increased plasma protein binding in epilepsy and trauma secondary to an increase in α_1-GP.

In liver failure, the free fraction may rise at the same time as the liver has decreased capacity to remove the drug. Therefore, an increase in free fraction does not always enhance clearance. Drug displacement interactions are especially important in liver dysfunction.

Decreased protein binding for high-extraction drugs will increase the apparent volume of distribution and the half-life. Whether the clearance of these drugs is affected will mainly depend on the effects of disease on liver perfusion. If liver perfusion decreases (and CL_{int} and V_d are stable) then free drug levels will rise, with the potential for increased toxicity. Toxicity is more likely to occur when hepatic function is severely compromised, when the drug has saturable metabolism, or when the drug has a narrow therapeutic range.

For low-extraction drugs the effects of liver disease are more difficult to predict. If there is no reduction in metabolic capacity, any increase
in free drug (due to reduced protein binding) may be compensated for by
an increase in drug clearance, which will tend to reduce the total blood
concentration, leaving the amount of free drug largely unaltered. However, the additional free drug may also be redistributed, leading to an
increase in the drug half-life. Effects of clinical importance occur when
low-extraction drugs suffer decreased protein binding and reduced
metabolism. The net effect is higher free drug concentrations. The extent
to which a drug is protein-bound will need to be considered when interpreting plasma drug concentrations, as reported levels reflect total drug
concentration rather than free, pharmacologically active drug. Where protein binding is reduced, clinical toxicity may occur at lower total plasma
concentrations.

Water-soluble drugs will have a significant increase in their volumes of distribution in patients with ascites, possibly necessitating larger
loading doses. Changes in apparent volume of distribution affect the use
of single doses of drugs (e.g. loading doses), whereas changes in drug
clearance are relevant to chronic dosing.

Absorption

Bioavailability is the term used to describe both the speed and extent of
absorption (symbolised by F and k_a). Systemic bioavailability is a product of absorption and first-pass metabolism. Liver disease decreases first-
pass metabolism and so increases bioavailability.

Cirrhosis may lead to portosystemic shunts and decreased activity
of a number of important drug-metabolising enzymes, which will result
in increased bioavailability of orally administered flow-limited drugs.
The oral bioavailability of a number of drugs with intermediate to high
hepatic extraction ratios has indeed been shown to be significantly
increased in patients with liver cirrhosis. For instance, the bioavailability of the sedative agent clomethiazole is increased more than 10-fold in
patients with cirrhosis. The increase in bioavailability in combination
with the decreased systemic clearance of flow-limited drugs in patients
with cirrhosis may lead to substantial increases in 'area under the curve',
necessitating a reduction in the administered dose. Similarly, propranolol and verapamil show increased bioavailability owing to a decrease
first-pass metabolism.

Decreased plasma protein binding in chronic liver disease may
theoretically reduce the oral availability owing to an increase in hepatic

extraction. However, reduced intrinsic clearance and portosystemic shunting are much more important determinants of the hepatic first-pass effect in chronic liver disease than alterations in plasma protein binding.

Portal hypertension is associated with oedema and structural abnormalities of the mucosa of the small intestine. This results in impaired oral absorption of some drugs, for example furosemide.

Varices, particularly bleeding varices, may increase the absorption of drugs that would normally exhibit poor absorption.

Metabolism

For drugs eliminated by the liver, clearance of unbound drug is dependent upon metabolic enzyme activity or, less frequently, upon hepatobiliary transport activity. A reduction in absolute liver cell mass and/or a decrease in enzyme level or activity due to alteration in the function of surviving cells may lead to impaired metabolism of a number of drugs. In addition, as a result of sinusoidal capillarisation, the uptake of certain drugs and of oxygen across the capillarised endothelium may be impaired, which may contribute to reduced hepatic drug metabolism in chronic liver disease.

The degree of impaired metabolism of drugs in patients with chronic liver disease varies from patient to patient and depends on the type of metabolic reaction involved. Oxidative metabolic reactions (catalysed by a large number of cytochrome P450 isoenzymes) appear to be more affected by chronic liver disease compared to glucuronidation. A study has shown that in human liver disease there is upregulation of the enzyme responsible for drug glucuronidation in the remaining viable hepatocytes. Chronic liver disease may have a variable effect on each of the individual cytochrome P450 isoenzymes.

Extrahepatic organs such as gut wall, kidney, lung, etc. provide an important contribution to the overall metabolism of drugs. Systemic clearance of propofol largely exceeds liver blood flow; this is because in chronic liver disease extrahepatic metabolism may compensate, at least in part, for the impaired metabolism of the drug by hepatic enzymes.

Plasma protein binding of drugs may be reduced in cholestasis owing to competition with bile salts for binding sites.

Biliary excretion

Chemical structure, polarity and molecular weight are the important characteristics of a drug that determine its excretion in bile. Drugs normally excreted to a significant extent via the bile may accumulate in patients with obstruction of the common bile duct. In addition, biliary obstruction may lead to hepatocellular damage with impairment of metabolic drug clearance.

Renal excretion

Because of reduced muscle mass and impaired metabolism of creatine to creatinine in a number of patients with severe liver disease, estimations of creatinine clearance are misleading representation of true renal function.

The hepatorenal syndrome is the renal impairment that occurs secondarily to liver disease. Poor liver clearance of vasodilating substances results in diversion to blood flow from liver and kidneys to the periphery. Reduced renal blood flow activates the renin–angiotensin–aldosterone pathway and produces an inappropriate tubular reabsorption of sodium and water. Secondary hyperaldosteronism results and is further intensified by the failure of the cirrhotic liver to metabolise aldosterone. Aldosterone is also highly protein-bound and the free level is increased by concurrent hypoalbuminaemia.

Altered pharmacodynamics in liver disease

The altered pharmacodynamics in cirrhosis affects many drug groups, for example β-adrenoreceptor antagonists, diuretics, analgesics (centrally acting), anxiolytics and sedatives. A decreased therapeutic effect is observed with β-adrenoreceptor antagonists and diuretics. In advanced cirrhosis, a reduction in β-adrenoreceptor density has been found in mononuclear cells.

A reduced pharmacodynamic effect has been observed with regard to diuretics. However, owing to reduced hepatic clearance in cirrhosis, a higher concentration of the diuretic may reach the kidney, thereby offsetting pharmacodynamic alterations except in cirrhotics with diuretic-resistant ascites. In these patients, the reduced pharmacodynamic effect could be due to a reduction in both the number of nephrons and the maximum response per nephron.

In contrast to β-adrenoreceptor antagonists and diuretics, an enhanced therapeutic effect and cerebral effect is observed in cirrhotic patients with analgesics, anxiolytics and sedatives. Encephalopathy may be precipitated when therapeutic doses of these drugs are administered to patients with cirrhosis. Various hypotheses have been proposed to explain the increased sensitivity of cirrhotic patients to these drugs, including alterations in blood–brain barrier permeability facilitating drug cerebral uptake, an increased GABAergic tone, or an increased number of GABA receptors and benzodiazepine-binding receptor ligands.

Liver function assessment

Plasma levels of substances such as bilirubin, bile pigments, albumin, clotting factors and enzymes (e.g. alkaline phosphatase) have not proved to be useful in characterising liver function in relation to drug pharmacokinetics and correlation between these conventional liver tests and pharmacokinetic behaviour of individual drugs tends to be unreliable. Among patients with the same diagnosis, structural damage and functional change of the liver vary widely between individuals. An alternative to the measurement of these endogenous biochemical markers is to use the clearance of exogenously administered model substrates to measure the liver's ability to eliminate drugs by metabolism or biliary excretion.

Model drugs used as indicators of changed drug clearance

Probe drugs

Probe drugs are not widely used in routine clinical practice; they are mainly reserved for research studies of liver dysfunction. However, they are being incorporated into liver transplantation surgery, where early restoration of liver performance is prognostic. A probe is used to quantify changes in hepatic blood flow, uptake, biotransformation and excretion as well as drug half-life, clearance and product formation rates (Barstow and Samal, 1990).

Normal liver function tests are expected to show a change in functional status or reflect tissue injury due to lack of vitamins (e.g. B_6). However, they can be misleading, as they could merely be revealing a change in hepatocellular permeability that allows enzymes to leach into plasma.

The ideal probe drug should have the following properties (Barstow and Samal, 1990):

- Its elimination should be entirely by hepatic metabolism.
- It should have linear kinetics.
- Its metabolism should be independent of liver blood flow and protein binding.

- The enzymes involved should be known.
- It should be a substrate for several isoenzymes and reflect several different pathways with measurable, inactive metabolites.
- It should have no pharmacology at doses used.
- It should be nontoxic to patients with liver dysfunction and healthy controls.
- It should produce no interactions with drugs or environment (genetics, diet, nutrition, etc.).
- It should be administered orally with rapid and complete absorption.
- It should be measurable in blood, saliva, urine or breath.
- There should exists a simple analysis kit.

Phenazone (antipyrine)

The test comprises an oral dose (10 mg/kg) and calculation of systemic clearance of phenazone by measuring the urine concentration of the major metabolites 4-hydroxyphenazone and 3-hydroxymethylphenazone (Farrell and Zalunzny, 1984). Oral absorption of phenazone is good and elimination is entirely by hepatic cytochrome P450 oxygenase (Friedman and Keefe, 2002) isoenzymes (CYP 1A2, 1A1 and 2D6, 2b6, 2c, 3a4).

Phenazone is the most investigated model drug for demonstrating the effects of liver disease on drug metabolism. The test shows good correlation with overall metabolic function but takes a long time to perform (Barstow and Samal, 1990).

Phenazone comes closest to the ideal agent because liver metabolism is the main route of elimination and half-life/clearance is sensitive to liver dysfunction that alters oxidative processes. It has low plasma protein binding and a low extraction ratio. Although the half-life of phenazone is increased in liver failure, it does not clearly correlate with *in vitro* assessment of hepatic microsomal capacity. Clearance is significantly impaired in cirrhosis and chronic active hepatitis but less so in acute liver disease and obstructive jaundice. The production of the demethylated metabolite norphenazone has been linked to all types of liver dysfunction.

The disadvantages of the test are that the long serum half-life of phenazone requires multiple sampling. It cannot be used as a real-time acute marker because the test takes at least 24 h and cannot be repeated for a week owing to enzyme induction.

Phenazone metabolism is affected by age, diet, alcohol, smoking and environmental exposure. Latterly, salivary testing has been shown to be a good indicator of plasma levels.

Aminophenazone (aminopyrine)

The test comprises an oral dose of ^{14}C-labelled dimethylaminophenazone (aminophenazone). $^{14}CO_2$ is measured in the breath 2 h after this dose. Aminophenazone undergoes N-demethylation by hepatic mixed-function oxidase catalysed by P450 isoenzymes 1a2, 2c9, 3a4.

The elimination pathway for this agent is vitamin B_{12}- and folate-dependent and is altered by infection and thyroid dysfunction. As long as there is no folate deficiency or thyroid disturbance, demethylation is the rate-limiting step.

Aminophenazone has a low extraction ratio (Tanaka and Breimer, 1997) and low first-pass metabolism. The test is noninvasive and has high sensitivity and low cost, but it requires confinement and the use of a radioactive substance.

The excretion is reduced with cirrhosis and acute liver disease (alcoholic hepatitis), but it is a poor indicator of cholestasis and extra-hepatic obstruction.

Caffeine clearance

Saliva or serum levels are determined following oral administration. The test is similar to the aminophenazone test but without the need for a radioisotope. Paraxanthine (1,7-dimethylxanthine) is the major metabolite and its production slows in cirrhosis. Cytochrome P450 1A2 is the major enzyme system (inducible by polycyclic aromatic hydrocarbons in cigarette smoke) (Barstow and Samal, 1990; Zimmerman, 1999).

The test is good for severe liver disease but not for mild dysfunction. Clearance decreases with age or by concurrent administration of cimetidine or oral contraceptives. Clearance increases with smoking.

Caffeine shows saturable metabolism across doses of 70–300 mg. The dose-dependence of the kinetics implies serial dosing and sampling with same dose (Chen *et al.*, 1990). The assay is an enzyme-modulated immunoassay. A graphical plot is made assuming $V_d = 0.61$ L/kg.

Saliva levels are unbound (normally 70% of total).

Erythromycin breath test

The demethylation of $[^{14}C]$erythromycin, monitored using $^{14}CO_2$ production, gives an indication of cytochrome P450 3A activity, which indicates ciclosporin clearance (Watkins *et al.*, 1990).

Galactose clearance

The oral test is done using [^{14}C]galactose, with measurement of breath $^{14}CO_2$. However, it is probably no better than standard liver function tests. Serial serum levels are determined between 20 and 50 min following IV or oral administration to estimate hepatic phosphorylation. [^{14}C]Galactose is distributed in extracellular water and is thus affected by volume changes and requires correction for renal elimination. Galactose has a high extraction ratio. Liver functional mass is assessed for blood levels over 500 mg/L. Clearance is reduced in acute and chronic liver disease and metastatic liver cancer but not in obstructive jaundice.

Indocyanine green

Indocyanine green (ICG) is a high-extraction drug used to assess liver blood flow. It is injected IV at 0.5 mg/kg IBW over 5 seconds with blood sampling over 1 h. It can only be used as a single-dose test because the second dose shows large variability owing to enzyme induction. In liver disease, hepatic extraction can reduce from 66% (in controls) to 33% of the ICG dose. As the blood levels fall, secondary binding sites outside the liver redistribute into plasma. Thus, late blood levels cannot indicate blood flow owing to third spacing.

Lidocaine

The test consists of the IV administration of 1 mg/kg of lidocaine. Fifteen minutes later, a plasma sample is taken to determine the level of monoethylglycinexylidide (MEGX) and glycinexylidide. Lidocaine undergoes sequential hepatic N-deethylation by cytochrome P450 isoenzyme 3A4 (Zimmerman, 1999).

Lidocaine has a high extraction ratio and is therefore sensitive to liver blood flow and cardiac output. MEGX can be measured by fluorescence polarisation immune assay in real time (Oellerich and Armstrong, 2001). The rapid turnaround is its key advantage. The test can be conducted during transplant surgery to monitor graft function and the inflammatory response to surgery. The test has been used to ascertain the need for transplantation (Tanaka et al., 2000), and to check the viability of donor liver allografts as well as early success of operation (Gao et al., 2000). It has been linked to Pugh–Child scoring and 6-month mortality in cirrhotic patients (Botta et al., 2003).

The MEGX test indicates the degree of cirrhosis but is unaffected by chronic active hepatitis. In cirrhosis the peak level may be delayed until 240 min post dose (Barstow and Samal, 1990). High bilirubin levels alter it and drugs metabolised by P450 3A4. It needs correction for cardiac function, age, weight and sex (males give higher results than females).

The MEGX test produces a better picture of hepatic functionality than does ICG (Oda *et al.*, 1995) or galactose (Barstow and Samal, 1990). It allows a rapid test, but interpatient variability means that it is not routine.

Modifications include reducing the dose to 0.5 mg/kg. This has been shown to be as good as the standard test (1 mg/kg) (Reichel *et al.*, 1997). Also, oral administration amplifies the IV information in indicating cirrhosis (Corpataux *et al.*, 2001). This is because in cirrhosis the first-pass metabolism will decrease and bioavailability will consequently increase. The assay method has also been changed to gas chromatography (GC) or high-pressure liquid chromatography (HPLC). This produces results that are specific for MEGX, but the GC and HPLC assays are more complicated.

Trimethadione (TMO)

This antiepileptic drug is rapidly and extensively metabolised by N-demethylation to dimethadione (DMO) using cytochrome P450 isoenzymes CYP 2c9, 2e1, 3a4. The parent drug has low plasma protein binding and first-order kinetics. Sampling is at 4 h post dose and elimination is independent of renal function (Barstow and Samal, 1990).

Metabolite-to-parent ratio gives an assessment of metabolic function. The DMO/TMO ratio is reduced in cirrhosis and chronic active hepatitis is but not affected by chronic persistent hepatitis or chronic active hepatitis. In disease states, the ratio shows good correlation with serum albumin, cholinesterase, ICG retention at 15 min, total bilirubin, total protein and prothrombin time, but not with aspartate aminotransferase (AST) or alanine aminotransferase (ALT).

No genetic polymorphism was detected in 1000 patients. The test is used to follow liver surgery because it has been shown that a DMO/TMO ratio >0.15 predicts survival. However, long-term use of TMO suppresses bone marrow, so it is used for short periods only.

Clinical case studies

These case studies are adapted and expanded from cases written by Gillian Cavell (Cavell, 1993).

CASE STUDY 4.1

An 81-year-old woman was admitted to hospital with a 3-week history of increasing jaundice and pale faeces and a 2-month history of darkening urine.

The liver function tests showed markedly raised serum total bilirubin, ALP (alkaline phosphatase) and GGT (gamma glutamyl transferase) with slightly elevated AST levels. Her plasma albumin level and prothrombin time were normal. A diagnosis of obstructive jaundice was made.

Comment on hepatic drug clearance in this patient

She has a normal plasma albumin level and is therefore likely to have normal hepatic synthetic function. It is usual to assume therefore that the patient should be able to conjugate bilirubin. An ALP level of more than three times the upper limit of normal in the presence of conjugated hyperbilirubinaemia is suggestive of posthepatic cholestasis. The elevation in serum bilirubin is due to the conjugated, water-soluble form. The onset of this obstructive jaundice has been relatively rapid and there is little or no hepatocellular damage reflected in a normal prothrombin time. It is unlikely that hepatic drug clearance in this patient will be adversely affected as hepatocellular function appears to be normal.

However, cholestasis can lead to the impaired absorption of lipid-soluble drugs and vitamins such as vitamin K. Vitamin K malabsorption results in defective coagulation. The plasma protein binding of drugs may be reduced in cholestasis owing to the competition with bile salts for plasma binding sites. Biliary excretion is often a significant route of elimination for drugs that are highly concentrated in bile. Patients with high GGT and ALP levels may experience a decrease in drug elimination via this route.

CASE STUDY 4.2

A 55-year-old woman was found to have deranged liver function tests on serum biochemistry. Liver biopsy was highly suggestive of chronic active hepatitis.

This patient has hepatocellular jaundice with a raised AST and elevated prothrombin time demonstrating acute hepatitis. In addition, her ALP and GGT are raised, indicating that the hepatitis has progressed to involve a cholestatic component. Her serum bilirubin is raised, which could be due to reduced

→

CASE STUDY 4.2 (continued)

conjugation or the secondary cholestatic effects. Her serum albumin level is low, indicating long-standing disease and reduced synthetic function.

Comment on hepatic drug clearance in this patient

Drug handling in this patient is likely to be altered due to a reduction in hepatocellular function. The half-lives of drugs that depend on the metabolic capacity of the liver for their clearance are likely to be increased in this patient. These drugs should be used in reduced doses to avoid the risk of accumulation and potential toxicity. Usually a dosage reduction of 50% is made for drugs given parenterally or for low-clearance drugs given orally. Drugs with a high hepatic extraction ratio administered orally should be used with caution because, while their clearance is blood flow-dependent, they do require some hepatic function.

Since the patient has a prolonged prothrombin time and therefore an increased risk of bleeding, drugs that alter platelet function or that may cause gastrointestinal bleeding should be avoided.

An increased level of toxins, such as bilirubin, can result in drugs being displaced from their binding sites, leading to an increased concentration of free drug. Additionally, a reduction in the serum albumin level will result in higher free drug concentrations. However, systemic bioavailability will depend on the capacity of the liver to metabolise the drug.

 CASE STUDY 4.3

A 53-year-old man with known alcoholic liver disease was admitted having been found collapsed at home. He was visibly jaundiced and showed other signs of chronic liver disease including spider naevi and ascites.

The prolongation of the prothrombin time, reduction of serum albumin and grossly elevated serum bilirubin indicate severe chronic liver disease, which had been confirmed by the presence of cirrhosis on biopsy during a previous admission.

Comment on the hepatic drug clearance in this patient

Cirrhosis of the liver will result in reduced hepatic blood flow and, in severe cases, reduced hepatocyte function. The raised prothrombin time and reduced

→

CASE STUDY 4.3 (continued)

albumin seen in this patient suggest the latter. There may also be portosystemic shunting, which results in drugs bypassing the liver after absorption from the gastrointestinal tract. This results in drugs entering the systemic circulation in higher concentrations.

Drugs with a high hepatic extraction will have a significantly reduced clearance owing to poor liver blood flow and their bioavailability when administered orally will be increased. The dose of drugs with a high hepatic extraction given orally is usually reduced to 10–50% of the normal dose and the patient is monitored closely for therapeutic efficacy and manifestations of toxicity. Drugs with a low hepatic extraction administered orally and drugs administered parenterally will be affected by the reduced metabolic capacity of the liver and therefore a 50% reduction in dose of these drugs should also be made.

Consideration should also be given to the risk of precipitating hepatic encephalopathy in patients with severe, chronic liver disease. Because of this, drugs with sedative effects or drugs that may cause electrolyte disturbances should be used with caution.

The patient's prolonged prothrombin time will result in an increased risk of bleeding, and therefore drugs that alter platelet function or that may cause gastrointestinal bleeding should be avoided.

The increased level of toxins such as bilirubin, and the reduced concentration of serum albumin, will result in raised concentrations of free drug.

Additionally, drugs that are renally excreted and are distributed into the body water (e.g. gentamicin) may have an increased volume of distribution in patients with ascites and oedema, as in this patient. This may necessitate alterations to drug dosages, particularly for loading doses.

CASE STUDY 4.4

A 44-year-old woman was admitted for the control of her fits. The neurologists started her on phenytoin and carbamazepine.

Her liver function test results were normal apart from a mildly raised ALP suggestive of simple cholestasis. However, she also had an elevated GGT. A normal serum bilirubin excludes cholestasis. The GGT level is approaching twice the ALP level and therefore enzyme induction by drugs is most likely.

→

> **CASE STUDY 4.4** (continued)

Comment on the hepatic drug clearance in this patient
Barbiturates, anticonvulsants, tricyclic antidepressants and rifampicin may all cause elevations of GGT as a result of enzyme induction. These elevations, usually between 2 and 5 times the normal value, are reversible on withdrawing the treatment. Enzyme induction may result in the increased metabolism of other hepatically cleared drugs, thus reducing their pharmacological effect. The dose of the affected drug may need to be modified.

References/Further reading

Barstow L, Samal R E (1990). Liver function assessment by drug metabolism. *Pharmacotherapy* 10(4): 280–288.

Botta F, Giannini E, Romagnoli P, *et al.* (2003). MELD scoring system is useful for predicting prognosis in patients with liver cirrhosis and is correlated with residual liver function: a European study. *Gut* 52(1): 134–139.

Cavell G (1993). Drug handling in liver disease. *Pharm J* 250: 352–355.

Chen WSC, Murphy T, Smith M, Cooksley W, Halliday J, Powell L (1990). Dose-dependent pharmacokinetics of caffeine in humans: relevance as a test of quantitative liver function. *Clin Pharmacol Ther* 47: 516–524.

Corpataux J M, Munafo A, Buclin J, Biollaz J, Mosimann F (2001). A preliminary evaluation of the discriminatory power of the monoethylglycinexylidide formation test after intravenous and oral administration of lidocaine. *Transplant Proc* 30: 2557–2562.

Curry H (1974). *Drug Disposition and Pharmacokinetics*. Oxford: Blackwell Scientific.

Farrell G C, Zalunzny L (1984). Accuracy and clinical utility of simplified tests of antipyrine metabolism *Br J Clin Pharmacol* 18: 559–565.

Friedman L S, Keefe E B (2002). *Handbook of Liver Diseases*. New York: Churchill Livingstone.

Gao L, Ramazan I, Baker A B (2000). Potential use of pharmacological markers to quantitatively assess liver function during liver transplant surgery. *Anaesth Intensive Care* 28(4): 375–385.

Gibaldi M (1984). *Biopharmaceutics and Clinical Pharmacokinetics*, 3rd edn. Philadelphia: Lea and Febiger.

Oda Y, Kariya N, Nakamoto T, Nishi S, Asada A, Fujimori M (1995). The monoethylglycinexylidide test is more useful for evaluating liver function than indocyanine green test: case of a patient with remarkably decreased indocyanine green half-life. *Ther Drug Monit* 17(2): 207–210.

Oellerich M, Armstrong V W (2001). The megx test: a tool for the real-time assessment of hepatic function. *Ther Drug Monit* 23(2): 81–92.

Reichel C, Nacke A, Sudhop T, *et al.* (1997). The low-dose monoethylglycinexylidide test: assessment of liver function with fewer side-effects. *Hepatology* 25(6): 1323–1327.

Tanaka E, Breimer D D (1997). *In vivo* function tests of hepatic drug oxidising capacity in patients with liver disease. *J Clin Pharm Ther* 22: 237–249.

Tanaka E, Inomata S, Yasuhara H (2000). The clinical importance of conventional and quantitative liver function tests in liver transplantation. *J Clin Pharm Ther* 25(6): 411–419.

Verbeeck R K, Horsman Y (1998). Effect of hepatic insufficiency on pharmacokinetics and drug dosing. *Pharm World Sci* 20(5): 183–192.

Watkins P, Hamilton T. Annesley T, Ellis CN, Kolars J, Voorhees J. The erythromycin breath test as a predictor of cyclosporin blood levels. *Clin Ther* 48 120–129.

Widdop B (1985). *Therapeutic Drug Monitoring*. Edinburgh: Churchill Livingstone.

Zimmerman HJ (1999). *Hepatotoxicity*. Philadelphia: Lippincott Williams and Wilkins.

5

Clinical pharmacokinetics in the elderly

Chris Cairns

Aims and learning outcomes

After reading this chapter, readers should:

- Know the differences in drug handling in elderly people compared to younger people.
- Understand the reasons why these changes occur.
- Know the drugs for which these changes have clinical implications.
- Have a basic knowledge of how to manage the potential problems associated with these implications.

Introduction

In pharmacokinetic terms, the elderly are a vulnerable group for a number of reasons. The ageing process and frailty alter older peoples' ability to handle drugs. As will be outlined in this chapter, the majority of these changes lead to increased blood levels and/or tissue levels of drugs. The elderly are further compromised by the fact that pharmacodynamically they exhibit increased sensitivity to many drugs (Gordon and Preiksaitis, 1988), but particularly those affecting the central nervous system.

Many drug interactions have clinical consequences as a result of a pharmacokinetic change. Polypharmacy is common in elderly patients and interactions can compound the kinetic vulnerability. Poorer homeostatic mechanisms (Swift, 1977; McGarry *et al.*, 1983) also mean that the elderly are more likely to suffer morbidity and even mortality as a consequence of an enhanced adverse effect of a drug due to increased serum levels.

Many of the kinetic changes in the elderly occur because of reductions in elimination ability, which occur as a consequence of the ageing process on the liver and kidney. For some drugs, however, there are significant changes in their absorption and distribution in the elderly and these processes must not be overlooked.

Absorption

There are a number of pathological changes in the elderly that can affect absorption. These are summarised in Box 5.1. These changes can have effects on drug dissolution, and the rate and extent of absorption.

The amount of saliva is reduced in old age and in theory the rate of absorption of drugs administered by the buccal and sublingual routes, e.g. glyceryl trinitrate, may be reduced. This could increase the time to reach maximum level (t_{max}) and hence delay onset of action. The overall extent of absorption is not affected.

Although gastric pH increases with age, there is no evidence available to show that this affects absorption (Bhanthumnavin and Schuster, 1977). There is a decrease in gastric secretion volume. This, combined with weakened peristalsis and delayed gastric emptying, may reduce the rate of absorption of drugs (Bhanthumnavin and Schuster, 1977). It is unlikely, however, to affect the extent of absorption.

Ageing has the effect of increasing the atrophy of the intestinal epithelium, producing a reduction of the jejunal mucosal surface area (Castleden *et al.*, 1977). This results in a reduced surface area for drug absorption. In addition, in the elderly there are reductions in blood flow in the splanchnic area and the mesenteries. As most drugs are absorbed by passive diffusion, this reduction in absorptive surface and the reduced concentration gradient from the reduced blood flow results in a slower rate of absorption. This in turn causes a delay in reaching peak drug level ($C_{p,max}$). The extent of absorption is rarely, if ever, affected. Although theoretically an issue in the clinical situation, this effect does not appear to cause problems (Castleden *et al.*, 1977; Iber *et al.*, 1994). Even relatively poorly absorbed drugs, such as ampicillin, show little or no difference between young and elderly populations (Iber *et al.*, 1994).

Box 5.1   Changes in gastrointestinal function with age

- Reduced saliva production
- Increased gastric pH
- Reduced gastric secretions
- Delayed gastric emptying
- Decreased gastric surface area
- Decreased gastrointestinal motility
- Decreased active transport processes

The absorption of some drugs that are absorbed through active transport mechanisms is reduced, including that of iron, calcium and vitamin B_{12} (Bhanthumnavin and Schuster, 1977). These appear to be an exception, as few other drugs absorbed by active processes are affected.

One drug that does exhibit significantly altered absorption is levodopa, which is commonly used in the elderly to treat Parkinson's disease. Substantial mucosal metabolism of this drug occurs by the enzyme dopa decarboxylase. There is a substantial increase in the absorption of levodopa in the elderly, probably owing to a reduction in the amount of dopa decarboxylase. Elderly patients show a slightly higher peak plasma level ($C_{p,max}$) and a shorter time to peak (t_{max}) than healthy young subjects (Evans *et al.*, 1980). The same difference in $C_{p,max}$ is seen in elderly healthy subjects (Robertson *et al.*, 1989). Both of these studies (Evans *et al.*, 1980; Robertson *et al.*, 1989) showed that the extent of absorption was increased with significantly higher areas under the curve (AUCs) in both elderly healthy volunteers and patients.

Reduction of regional blood flow in older people can be caused by the replacement of tissue by connective tissue and fat (Anon, 1978). This may cause reductions in the rate of absorption following subcutaneous or intramuscular administration. There is no evidence, however, that this causes any significant clinical effects.

Distribution

Factors that can affect drug distribution in the elderly are summarised in Box 5.2. The two single most important factors are changes in body composition and protein binding.

As the body ages, there are significant changes in composition. Lean body mass declines by as much as 12–19% (Main, 1988). In contrast, adipose tissue increases by 14–35% as a proportion of total body weight. This occurs even in the absence of overt obesity. These changes are combined with a decrease in total body water. Because a drug's volume of distribution (V_d) is dependent on how it distributes into the body's aqueous and lipid phases, these changes will have a significant effect on drug distribution. This will be particularly significant if a drug is highly lipid-soluble, is distributed widely into muscle, or is largely confined to body water. Basic knowledge of kinetics tells us that $V_d = A/C_p$, where A is the amount of drug in the body and C_p is the plasma concentration. Changes in V_d due to changes in body composition will therefore lead to changes in serum concentration. Drugs with a low V_d, such as warfarin and

---

Box 5.2 Factors affecting drug distribution

Body composition changes	Increased adipose tissue
	Reduced body water
	Decreased muscle mass
Protein binding changes	Increased α_1-acid glycoprotein
	Decreased albumin
Reductions in systemic perfusion	Reduced cardiac output
	Increased vascular resistance
Increased permeability across blood–brain barrier	

---

gentamicin, are not widely distributed. Those with a large V_d, such as digoxin and amiodarone, are extensively distributed.

For fat-soluble drugs, in the elderly the V_d is increased owing to the increase in body fat. This has been demonstrated for diazepam (Klotz *et al.*, 1975), lidocaine (Nation *et al.*, 1977), thiopental, midazolam (Collier *et al.*, 1982) and clomethiazole. The adipose tissue acts as a reservoir for these drugs and an enhanced $t_{1/2}$ is also seen, resulting in a prolonged duration of action. The fact that ageing reduces metabolism has an additive effect on this. The V_d of diazepam is increased from 1.19 L/kg in young males to 1.65 L/kg in elderly males (Divoll *et al.*, 1983). Changes of a similar magnitude are found in females: 1.87 L/kg and 2.46 L/kg, respectively (Divoll *et al.*, 1983).

Older people are more sensitive to the central nervous system (CNS) effects of benzodiazepines even when there are no obvious pharmacokinetic changes. Although this may be due to increased receptor sensitivity or response, it may also be due to increased distribution of the drug into the brain (Gordon and Preiksaitis, 1988).

Water-soluble drugs, conversely, tend to experience a reduction in V_d, resulting in higher serum levels. This can be found in the case of gentamicin, ethanol, theophylline and cimetidine.

Digoxin, although water-soluble, has a relatively high V_d. This is due to widespread distribution into muscle. The reduction in muscle mass in older people means there is a significant reduction in digoxin's V_d (Cusack *et al.*, 1979; Hanratty *et al.*, 2000). The clinical consequence of this is that loading doses have to be substantially reduced in the elderly.

Two circulating proteins are altered in old age that have significant effects on drug handling. Serum albumin is reduced while α_1-acid glycoprotein is increased (Reidenberg and Erill, 1986). The effects of these changes can be complex. They are further complicated in renal and hepatic diseases, as these conditions have effects on circulating endogenous products and protein formation. Poor nutrition and debilitation will further complicate the picture.

In the elderly, serum albumin is decreased by around 10–13% (Wallace and Verbeeck, 1987). In general, acidic drugs tend to bind to albumin and so are more likely to be affected. Therefore, it is likely that drugs such as cimetidine, furosemide (Kelly *et al.*, 1974), nonsteroidal anti-inflammatory drugs (NSAIDs) and sulfonylureas will be affected. Increases in free fractions of naproxen, diflunisal and salicylates have been found in the elderly (Wallace and Verbeeck, 1987). It is thought that protein binding changes may be a contributing factor in the increased toxicity of NSAIDs seen in older people (Solomon and Gurwitz, 1997).

Highly protein-bound drugs such as warfarin and phenytoin are also likely to be affected. Phenytoin is an excellent example of the complexity of these changes in old age. Phenytoin is highly protein bound. The reduction in serum albumin means that a higher proportion of an administered dose exists in free form in the plasma (Perucca, 1984). However, bound drug is not available for distribution or elimination, while the free fraction is. The fact that there are increased amounts of free fraction available for elimination results in increased clearance (Bach *et al.*, 1981). Dosage need not be altered as tissue levels remain unchanged, but serum levels tend to be reduced and this must be reflected when interpreting drug levels. A number of refinements have been made since the original Winter–Tozer equation was proposed (Tozer and Winter, 1992).

$$[PHT]_{normalised} = [PHT]_{observed} \times \frac{44}{[ALB]}$$

where $[PHT]_{normalised}$ is the adjusted serum phenytoin level as in a non-hypoalbuminaemic patient, $[PHT]_{observed}$ the actual phenytoin level in the hypoalbuminaemic patient and $[ALB]$ the serum albumn in g/L.

More recently Anderson *et al.* (1997) have proposed a modified version:

$$[PHT]_{normalised} = \frac{[PHT]_{measured}}{0.25 \times [ALB] + 0.1}$$

Again where $[PHT]_{normalised}$ is the adjusted serum phenytoin level as in a nonhypoalbuminaemic patient, $[PHT]_{measured}$ the actual phenytoin level in the hypoalbuminaemic patient and $[ALB]$ the serum albumin in g/dL. Care must be taken when using the modified equation as it utilises the US units for measuring albumin (g/dL). However, it can be used as long as the g/L value is converted to g/dL before the calculation is carried out.

Metabolism

The majority of drug metabolism takes place in the liver, although there is limited metabolism in the lungs and kidneys. Some drugs including suxamethonium and atracurium are metabolised in the blood. In the elderly, hepatic blood flow is reduced by up to 40% (Tregaskis and Stevenson, 1990) and this significantly reduces the delivery of drug to the liver. The consequence of this is reduced metabolism, leading to longer half-lives and increases in C_p.

Four major processes each have an effect on the rate of metabolism of a drug: first-pass mechanism, hepatic blood flow, extraction from the blood, and metabolic capacity. The effect of each of these in the elderly depends on the properties of individual drugs.

The first-pass mechanism affects a number of lipid-soluble drugs. Metabolism occurs as these drugs are transported via the portal circulation, following absorption but before reaching the general circulation. The reduction in blood flow results in increases in systemic bioavailability. For some drugs the proportion of drug remaining after first-pass metabolism can be low, 5–10% of the dose, so that small decreases in first-pass metabolism can lead to significant increases in bioavailability. Significant changes in blood pressure reduction have been shown, which are due to increased bioavailability of nifedipine (Durnas *et al.*, 1990). Other drugs for which there is a high first-pass effect that can affect bioavailability include propranolol (Castledon *et al.*, 1975), labetalol, verapamil and the nitrates. Increased bioavailability can be expected with these drugs.

Metabolism is the main route of elimination for many drugs. This process is affected in the elderly by reduced hepatic blood flow as previously outlined, and the metabolic capacity of the liver. This capacity is reduced significantly in old age, by up to 60% (Solomon and Gurwitz, 1997), and this will lead to higher blood levels and longer $t_{1/2}$ for many drugs. Reductions in metabolic capacity have been shown to increase levels of NSAIDs (Solomon and Gurwitz, 1997), phenytoin (Bach *et al.*, 1981) and narcotic analgesics. Diazepam's half-life increases dramatically with age up to 79 h (range 37–169 h) (Salzman *et al.*, 1983). The half-life of midazolam is similarly extended in the elderly (Servin *et al.*, 1987).

The reduction in hepatic blood flow, on the other hand is the main factor in the reduced metabolism of hypnotics and antipsychotics. Clozapine levels increase with age in both men and women, probably owing to reduced hepatic clearance (Kurz *et al.*, 1998). Clomethiazole has been shown to have its half-life prolonged more than twofold in the elderly (Nation *et al.*, 1976, 1977b). This can result in serum levels of up to five times normal. Lisinopril has serum levels and AUCs in the elderly that are double those seen in younger patients (Langtry and Markham, 1997; Rush and Lyle, 1988).

Determining the likely effect of ageing on drug metabolism is not easy as there is no simple reliable marker of liver function in the same way that creatinine can be used for renal function. The fact that the liver's metabolic function is a combination of hepatic blood flow, the liver's ability to extract the drug from the circulation, and metabolic capacity further complicate matters. There are some general principles that can be applied, however. Drugs can be divided into three groups depending on the liver's ability to extract them from the circulation: high, medium or low extraction ratio.

Drugs with a high hepatic extraction ratio have a high proportion of the drug removed from the circulation in a single pass through the liver. The consequence of this is that the metabolism of these drugs is highly dependent on liver blood flow (Wilkinson and Shand, 1975). In the elderly, the clearance of these drugs will be reduced both by first pass and the reduced hepatic blood flow. Drugs particularly affected include morphine, propranolol and a number of the calcium antagonists. In the elderly, some calcium antagonists may have levels elevated 1.5–2 times those found in the general population (Durnas *et al.*, 1990). Lidocaine is metabolised to an active metabolite, monoethylglycinexylidide (MEGX), which is active but less potent (Halkin *et al.*, 1975). During continuous epidural infusion the plasma MEGX to lidocaine ratio is higher in younger compared to older women (Fukada *et al.*, 2000). As this mode of administration bypasses the first-pass mechanism, this shows a slowing in the metabolic rate of lidocaine. The authors speculated that this may be due to decreased cytochrome P450 3A4 activity or reduction in hepatic blood flow.

Drugs with a low hepatic extraction ratio, conversely, have a small proportion removed during their pass through the liver. Hence changes in hepatic blood flow have minimal effects on them. The intrinsic metabolic capacity of the liver will be the most important factor. As outlined above, this can be reduced by up to 60% in old age (Solomon and Gurwitz, 1997). Although it is recognised that liver metabolic capacity in old age is reduced, there are few conclusive studies on the effects of ageing on specific liver enzymes. There is a general acceptance that enzymes responsible for Phase I processes such as oxidation are affected more by old age compared to the Phase II enzymes responsible for conjugation processes. The demethylation of amitriptyline (Dawling *et al.*, 1982), of imipramine

(Abernethy *et al.*, 1985) and of thioridazine (Cohen and Sommer, 1988) are all decreased in the elderly.

It is not a given that drugs eliminated by the liver have reduced clearance in the elderly. Theophylline has been shown to have similar clearance in elderly patients compared to otherwise healthy young asthmatics (Nielsen-Kudsk *et al.*, 1978) despite a reduction in demethylation (Antal *et al.*, 1981). The latter study has shown a reduced clearance, but this was very slight. The small but significant proportion of digoxin eliminated by metabolism (16%) does not seem to be affected by age (Hui *et al.*, 1994).

Elimination

As one ages, renal function decreases. Between the ages of 20 and 80 years, the kidney decreases in size by about 20%, with a loss of around 30% of functioning glomeruli. This results in a loss of up to half of renal function (Davies and Shock, 1950). This is seen as a reduction in glomerular filtration rate (GFR). Many drugs are eliminated unchanged solely or mainly by renal excretion. The relationship between drug elimination and GFR means that drugs that are predominantly removed from the body by this route will exhibit altered kinetics. The half-life of chlorpropamide increases from 25–48 h (Ciechanowski *et al.*, 1999) in younger patients to 99 h in elderly diabetics (Arrigoni *et al.*, 1987), for example. Tramadol appears to show some relationship between increasing serum levels and reductions in creatinine clearance, and lower doses should be used in the elderly (Ofoegbu, 1984). The clearance of furosemide is decreased in the elderly (Chaturvedi *et al.*, 1987). However, furosemide is eliminated both renally and hepatically and it is not known whether this reduction is due to hepatic or renal changes.

In general, reduced clearance will be reflected in extended half-life (with corresponding reductions in elimination rate constant) and increased serum levels. Gentamicin and digoxin are two commonly used drugs, both with a narrow therapeutic window, that are eliminated in this way. Unless dosage is adjusted in the elderly, the reduced clearance will lead to accumulation and toxicity. There is a clear relationship between GFR and the elimination rate of these drugs (Doherty and Kane, 1973; Lackner and Birge, 1990). There are also reductions in active tubular secretion and reabsorption, although the clinical significance of these is unknown. The half-life of gentamicin in elderly patients (>70 years) is approximately 4.1 h compared with 2.8 h in younger patients (<55 years) (Lackner and Birge, 1990).

Although serum creatinine is a very good marker of renal function because it has a proportional relationship with GFR, it has major limitations in the elderly. The serum creatinine level is a balance between its renal clearance and its production as a consequence of muscle turnover. Elderly people have less muscle mass, so the production of creatinine is reduced in addition to the reduced renal clearance. Hence, elderly people usually have a serum creatinine in the normal range despite significantly reduced renal function (Rowe *et al.*, 1976). However, GFR and tubular secretion decrease at a constant rate with increasing age. This means that drug elimination decreases in direct proportion with creatinine clearance. The use of creatinine clearance to predict the effect of age-related deterioration in renal function is much more reliable than using serum creatinine. Equations such as that of Cockcroft and Gault (Cockcroft and Gault, 1976) for calculating creatinine clearance are reliable for the majority of elderly patients as they take into account both body mass and age as well as renal function.

As long as the additional effects of ageing on V_d and other factors such as protein binding are taken into account when appropriate, the main principles of managing drug dosage in renal impairment, discussed in Chapter 3, can be applied. However, as in the case of metabolism, changes do not always occur. In a single-dose study the peak plasma concentration, AUC and half-life of captopril in older volunteers were similar to those observed in younger volunteers (Creasey *et al.*, 1986).

The effect of reduced renal function on the elimination of drug metabolites must also be considered. Many metabolites, including some that are active, are removed by renal excretion. Accumulation of renally cleared active metabolites, such as morphine-6-glucuronide, morphine-3-glucuronide (Glare and Walsh, 1991) and laudanosine (from atracurium), can lead to toxicity (Nigrovic and Banoub, 1992). Midazolam metabolites, many of which are active, can accumulate in patients with poor renal function (de Wildt *et al.*, 2001).

Other factors

Acute illness can lead to compromised handling of a number of drugs. For example, congestive cardiac failure (CCF) and acute infection both reduce the elimination of theophylline (Hendeles *et al.*, 1995). Renal function can also be reduced further in patients with acute pneumonia or following an acute myocardial infarction. Elderly patients on drugs with narrow therapeutic windows, such as theophylline or digoxin, may develop toxicity due to elevated levels, during an acute illness, despite previously having had stable levels in the normal range. Furosemide, conversely, is poorly absorbed in patients with decompensated CCF and may be ineffective (Vasko *et al.*, 1985).

Similarly, it must be remembered that in addition to the age-related changes discussed here, elderly patients suffer the same diseases and are treated with the same drugs as younger patients. This means that any effects on drug handling from pathology and/or drug interactions will have an additive effect to the already existing age-related changes. The fact that elderly patients have reduced homeostasis (Swift, 1977) and show increased sensitivity for some drugs (Gordon and Preiksaitis, 1988) will exacerbate this situation further.

Conclusions

The older patient handles many drugs differently from younger patients. These changes can affect any of the processes involved in drug handling. The usual consequence, but not always, is an increased serum level leading to toxicity. All medicines should be used with caution in older people, but particularly those medicines with a narrow therapeutic window.

Clinical case studies

CASE STUDY 5.1

Mr J.K. is an 86-year-old man who has developed a ventricular arrhythmia following an angioplasty, which is proving resistant to both lidocaine and amiodarone. Beta blockers are contraindicated as he has chronic obstructive pulmonary disease (COPD). Flecainide is considered as an appropriate third-line agent. He has a normal serum creatinine of 89 mmol/L and weighs 58 kg.

Does he require a dose reduction for his flecainide?
Flecainide is primarily excreted by the kidney and its dose requires to be reduced in renal impairment. Flecainide has significant toxicity that is serum level-related. Mr J.K.'s serum creatinine is in the normal range but, as he is elderly, this may not be reflective of normal renal function. Renal function deteriorates with age and elderly patients frequently have a reduced muscle mass. Applying the equation of Cockcroft and Gault to Mr J.K.'s indices gives an estimated creatinine clearance of 44 mL/min, less than half of normal renal function. This level of impairment is considered minor, but the maximum initial dose of flecainide recommended is 100 mg daily rather than 100 mg twice a day (200 mg daily).

CASE STUDY 5.2

Benzodiazepines like diazepam have an increased volume of distribution (V_d) in the elderly. For example the V_d of diazepam is 1.19 L/kg in young males but increases to 1.65 L/kg in elderly males. At a ward round, one of your SHO colleagues asks you why you advised a reduced dose for an elderly patient, when normally an increase in V_d means that an increased dose is required.

Discussion
For fat-soluble drugs such as diazepam, the V_d in older people is increased owing to the increase in body fat. This adipose tissue acts as a reservoir for these drugs and causes a prolonging of half-life ($t_{1/2}$) resulting in a prolonged duration of action. Ageing also reduces metabolism of benzodiazepines, resulting in reduced clearance, which further increases the half-life.

In addition, older people are more sensitive to the CNS effects of benzodiazepines even when there are no obvious pharmacokinetic changes. Although this may be due to increased receptor sensitivity or response, it may also be due to increased distribution of the drug into the brain.

Answer
Single pharmacokinetic changes in the elderly must not be viewed in isolation but should be seen in the context of overall pharmacokinetic changes. Any pharmacodynamic changes must also be considered. As the net effect is reduced clearance and increased serum levels, coupled to increased sensitivity, it is appropriate to reduce the dosage of diazepam in elderly patients.

CASE STUDY 5.3

Mrs A.D. is a 79-year-old lady with a history of COPD and ischaemic heart disease (IHD), both of which are normally well controlled on drug treatment. Her usual prescription is:

Salbutamol inhaler:	*2 puffs q.d.s.*
Ipratropium inhaler:	*2 puffs q.d.s.*
Aminophylline SR:	*450 mg b.d.*
Furosemide:	*40 mg mane*
Aspirin:	*75 mg mane*

$\rightarrow$

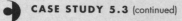 **CASE STUDY 5.3** (continued)

Simvastatin:	*20 mg nocte*
Ramipril:	*10 mg mane*

She presents to A&E in considerable distress, being 'unable to catch her breath'. On examination she has severe pitting oedema in both lower legs and raised jugular venous pulse, and chest auscultation reveals significant fluid accumulation in both lungs, which is confirmed by chest radiography. A diagnosis of acute pulmonary oedema due to her ischaemic heart failure is made. It is decided to treat her with furosemide.

What pharmacokinetic considerations are necessary?

There are two principal considerations. The absorption of furosemide is significantly reduced in acute heart failure owing to congestion in splanchnic and hepatic blood vessels. In many circumstances oral furosemide is ineffective. Increasing the oral dose rarely improves this situation. The drug requires to be given parenterally, usually intravenously. Rapid injection of furosemide is associated with damage to the ear and can cause both dizziness and deafness. As older people usually have a loss in auditory acuity and are at risk of falls, it is important to avoid causing either or both of these. The dose should be given slowly, certainly no faster than 4 mg/min.

The second consideration is theophylline, the active component of aminophylline. In congestive heart failure theophylline is less well metabolised and can reach toxic levels. Mrs A.D.'s theophylline level should be measured and dosage adjustment made if necessary. It is important to re-assess Mrs A.D.'s theophylline requirements when her acute condition has resolved and make the necessary adjustments.

 CASE STUDY 5.4

You have been forwarded Mr J.'s phenytoin level, which was taken at his routine 6-monthly visit to his neurologist. The level is 7.6 mg/L which is subtherapeutic. The doctor is concerned that although Mr J. has not had a recent seizure, he is 76 years old and is possibly at risk. As Mr J. still drives, the doctor feels that an increase in dose would be in order. The doctor is aware that increases in phenytoin dose must be carefully done owing to the capacity-limited kinetics it exhibits and so refers this adjustment to the pharmacy TDM service.

→

CASE STUDY 5.4 (continued)

What further information do you require and what adjustment is necessary?
In addition to the usual information such as dosing history, dose, and timing of levels, it is important in the elderly (and other patients with significant pathology) to obtain a recent albumin level. In the elderly, serum albumin is frequently reduced. As phenytoin is significantly bound to albumin, any reduction in serum albumin will lead to a reduced serum level. However, owing to distribution and elimination of unbound phenytoin, free levels of phenytoin are unaffected and the concentration at receptor sites is unchanged.

Mr J. has a serum albumin of 32 g/L, which is considerably below normal. The equation

$$C_{normalised} = C_{observed} \times \frac{44}{observed\ albumin}$$

can be used to adjust the level in a hypoalbuminaemic patient. $C_{normalised}$ is what the serum phenytoin level would be if the patient did not have hypoalbuminaemia and $C_{observed}$ is the actual level in the hypoalbuminaemic patient. Although there is some variation in how applicable this equation is, it will give a good guide to whether dosage adjustment is necessary. Applying this to Mr J. gives

$$\begin{aligned} C_{normalised} &= 7.6 \times 44/32 \\ &= 7.6 \times 1.375 \\ &= 10.45\ mg/L \quad (10.5\ mg/L\ to\ one\ decimal\ place) \end{aligned}$$

This level of 10.5 mg/L is at the bottom end of the effective therapeutic range, so Mr J.'s seemingly low phenytoin level adjusts to be within the effective therapeutic range. As he has no history of fits, it would be unwise to change his dosage. Not only is he unlikely to derive any benefit, but dosage adjustment with phenytoin is fraught with difficulty owing to its saturation kinetics and could be made toxic, especially if his hypoalbuminaemia is not taken into consideration. This case also reinforces the lesson that it is the patient who should be treated and not the number obtained from a laboratory result.

References/Further reading

Abernethy D R, Greenblatt D J, Shader R I (1985). Imipramine and desipramine disposition in the elderly. *J Pharmacol Exp Ther* 232: 183–188.

Anon (1978). Drug use in the elderly: a review of problems and special considerations [Editorial]. *Drugs* 16: 358–382.

Anderson G S, Pak C, Doane K W *et al.* (1997). Revised Winter–Tozer equation for normalizing phenytoin concentrations in trauma and elderly patients. *Ann Pharmacother* 31: 279–284.

Antal E J, Kramer P A, Mercik S A *et al.* (1981). Theophylline kinetics in advanced age. *Br J Clin Pharmacol* 12: 637–646.

Armour D, Cairns C, eds. (2002). *Medicines in the Elderly*. London: Pharmaceutical Press.

Arrigoni L, Fundak G, Horn J *et al.* (1987). Chlorpropamide pharmacokinetics in young healthy adults and older diabetic patients. *Clin Pharm* 6: 162–164.

Bach B, Molholm-Hansen J, Kamomann J P *et al.* (1981). Disposition of antipyrine and phenytoin correlated with age and liver volume in man. *Clin Pharmacokinet* 6: 389–386.

Bhanthumnavin K, Schuster M (1977). Ageing and gastrointestinal function. In: Finch C E, Hayflick L, eds. *Handbook of the Biology of Ageing*. New York: Van Nostrand Reinhold, 709–723.

Castleden C M, Kaye C M, Parson R L (1975). The effect of age on plasma levels of propranolol and practolol in man. *Br J Clin Pharmacol* 2: 303.

Castleden C M, Volans C N, Raymond K (1977). The effect of ageing on drug absorption from the gut. *Age Ageing* 6: 138–143.

Chaturvedi P R, O'Donnell J P, Nicholas J M *et al.* (1987). Steady state absorption kinetics and pharmacodynamics of furosemide in congestive heart failure. *Int J Clin Pharmacol Ther Toxicol* 25: 123–128.

Ciechanowski K, Borowiak K S, Potocka B A *et al.* (1999). Chlorpropamide toxicity with survival despite 27-day hypoglycemia. *J Toxicol Clin Toxicol* 37: 869–871.

Cockcroft D W, Gault M H (1976). Prediction of creatinine clearance from serum creatinine. *Nephron* 16: 31–41.

Cohen B M, Sommer B R (1988). Metabolism of thioridazine in the elderly. *J Clin Psychopharmacol* 8: 336–339.

Collier P, Kawar P, Gamble J A S *et al.* (1982). Influence of age on pharmacokinetics of midazolam. *Br J Clin Pharmacol* 13: 602P.

Creasey W A, Funke P T, McKinstry D N *et al.* (1986). Pharmacokinetics of captopril in elderly healthy male volunteers. *J Clin Pharmacol* 26: 264–268.

Cusack B, Horgan J, Kelly J G *et al.* (1979). Digoxin in the elderly: pharmacokinetic consequences of old age. *Clin Pharmacol Ther* 25: 772–776.

Davies D F, Shock N W (1950). Age changes in glomerular filtration rate, effective renal plasma flow and tubular excretory capacity in adult males. *J Clin Invest* 29: 496–501.

Dawling S, Lynn K, Rosser R *et al.* (1982). Nortryptiline metabolism in chronic renal failure: metabolic elimination. *Clin Pharmacol Ther* 32: 322–329.

de Wildt S N, Kearns G L, Hop W C J *et al.* (2001). Pharmacokinetics and metabolism of intravenous midazolam in preterm infants. *Clin Pharmacol Ther* 70: 525–531.

Divoll M, Greenblatt D J, Ochs H R *et al.* (1983). Absolute bioavailability of oral and intramuscular diazepam, effects of age and sex. *Anesth Analg* 62: 1–8.

Doherty J E, Kane J J (1973). Clinical pharmacology and therapeutic use of digitalis glycosides. *Drugs* 6: 182–221.

Durnas C, Loi C, Cusack B (1990). Hepatic drug metabolism and ageing. *Clin Pharmacokinet* 19: 359–389.

Evans M A, Triggs E J, Broe G A *et al.* (1980). Systemic availability of orally administered L-dopa in the elderly Parkinson patient. *Eur J Clin Pharmacol* 17: 215–221.

Fukuda T, Kakiuchi Y, Miyabe M *et al.* (2000). Plasma lidocaine, monoethyl-glycinexylidide, and glycinexylidide concentrations after epidural administration in geriatric patients. *Reg Anesth Pain Med* 25: 268–273.

Glare P A, Walsh T D (1991). Clinical pharmacokinetics of morphine. *Ther Drug Monit* 13: 1–23.

Gordon M, Preiksaitis H G (1988). Drugs and the ageing brain. *Geriatrics* 43: 69–78.

Halkin H, Meffin P, Melmon K L *et al.* (1975). Influence of congestive heart failure on blood levels or lidocaine and its active monodeethylated metabolite. *Clin Pharmacol Ther* 17: 669–676.

Hanratty C G, McGlinchey P, Johnston G D *et al.* (2000). Differential pharmacokinetics of digoxin in elderly patients. *Drugs Aging* 17: 353–362.

Hendeles L, Jenkins J, Temple R (1995). Revised FDA labeling guideline for theophylline oral dosing forms. *Pharmacotherapy* 15: 409–427.

Hui J, Geraets D R, Chandrasekaran A *et al.* (1994). Digoxin disposition in elderly humans with hypochlorhydria. *J Clin Pharmacol* 34: 734–741.

Iber F L, Murphy P, Connor E S (1994). Age-related changes in the gastrointestinal system. Effects on drug therapy. *Drugs Aging* 5: 34–38.

Kelly M R, Cutler R E, Forrey A W *et al.* (1974). Pharmacokinetics of orally administered furosemide. *Clin Pharmacol Ther* 15: 178–186.

Klotz U, Avant G R, Hoyumpa A *et al.* (1975). The effects of age and liver disease in the distribution and elimination of diazepam in adult man. *J Clin Invest* 55: 347–359.

Kurz M, Hummer M, Kemmler G *et al.* (1998). Long-term pharmacokinetics of clozapine. *Br J Psychiatry* 173: 341–344.

Lackner T E, Birge S (1990). Accuracy of pharmacokinetic dose determination of gentamicin in geriatric patients. *D IC P Ann Pharmacother* 24: 29–32.

Langtry H D, Markham A (1997). Lisinopril: a review of its pharmacology and clinical efficacy in elderly patients. *Drugs Aging* 10: 131–166.

Main A (1988). Elderly patients and their drugs. *Pharm J* 240: 537–539.

McGarry K, Laher M, Fitzgerald D *et al.* (1983). Baroreflex function in elderly hypertensives. *Hypertension* 5: 763–766.

Nation R L, Laeroyd B, Barber J *et al.* (1976). The pharmacokinetics of chlormethiazole following intravenous administration in the aged. *Eur J Clin Pharmacol* 10: 407–415.

Nation R L, Triggs E J, Selig M (1977a). Lidocaine kinetics in cardiac patients and elderly subjects. *Br J Clin Pharmacol* 4: 439–448.

Nation R L, Vine J, Triggs E J *et al.* (1977b). Plasma level of chlormethiazole and two metabolites after oral administration to young and aged human subjects. *Eur J Clin Pharmacol* 12: 137–145.

Nielsen-Kudsk F, Magnussen I, Jakobsen P (1978). Pharmacokinetics of theophylline in then elderly patients. *Acta Pharmacol Toxicol* 42: 226–234.

Nigrovic V, Banoub M (1992). Pharmacokinetic modelling of a parent drug and its metabolite atracurium and laudanosine. *Clin Pharmacokinet* 22: 396–408.

Ofoegbu R O (1984). Report on a clinical trial with tramadol hydrochloride (Tramal) in the prevention of post-operative pain. *Curr Ther Res* 36: 436–444.

Perucca E (1984). Free level monitoring of antiepileptic drugs: clinical usefulness and case studies. *Clin Pharmacokinet* 9: 71–78.

Reidenberg M M, Erill S, eds. (1986). *Drug–Protein Binding*. New York: Praeger, 163–171.

Robertson D R, Wood N D, Everest H *et al.* (1989).The effect of age on the pharmacokinetics of levodopa administered alone and in the presence of carbidopa. *Br J Clin Pharmacol* 28: 61–69.

Rowe J W, Andres R, Tobin J D *et al.* (1976). The effect of age on creatinine clearance in man: a cross sectional and longitudinal study. *J Gerontol* 31: 155–163.

Rush J E, Lyle P A (1988). Safety and tolerability of lisinopril in older hypertensive patients. *Am J Med* 85(supplement 3B): 55–59.

Salzman C, Shader R I, Greenblatt D J *et al.* (1983). Long vs. short half-life benzodiazepines in the elderly: kinetics and clinical effects of diazepam and oxazepam. *Arch Gen Psychiatry* 40: 293–297.

Servin F, Enriquez I, Foumet M *et al.* (1987). Pharmacokinetics of midazolam used as an intravenous induction agent for patients over 80 years of age. *Eur J Anaesthesiol* 4: 1–7.

Solomon D H, Gurwitz J H (1997). Toxicity of nonsteroidal anti-inflammatory drugs in the elderly: is advanced age a risk factor? *Am J Med* 102: 208–215.

Swift C G (1977). Pharmacodynamics: changes in homeostatic mechanisms, receptor and target organ sensitivity in the elderly. *BMJ* 1: 10–12.

Tozer T N, Winter M E (1992). In: Evans W E, Schentag J J, Jusko W J, eds. *Applied Pharacokinetics: Principles of Therapeutic Drug Monitoring*, 3rd edn. Vancouver: Applied Therapeutics.

Tregaskis B F, Stevenson I H (1990). Pharmacokinetics in old age. *Br Med Bull* 46: 9–21.

Vasko M R, Brown-Cartwright D, Knochel J P *et al.* (1985). Furosemide absorption altered in decompensated congestive heart failure. *Ann Intern Med* 102: 314–318.

Wallace S M, Verbeeck R V (1987). Plasma protein binding of drugs in the elderly. *Clin Pharmacokinet* 12: 41–72.

Wilkinson G R, Shand D G (1975). A physiological approach to hepatic drug metabolism. *Clin Pharmacol Ther* 18: 277–390.

6

Aminoglycosides

Neil A Caldwell

Aims and learning outcomes

The aim of this chapter is to understand clinical pharmacokinetic handling of aminoglycoside therapy. After completing this chapter readers should be able to:

- Take responsibility for assessing and meeting the drug-related needs of patients receiving aminoglycoside therapy.
- Assess the appropriateness, or otherwise, of aminoglycoside dosing regimens based on population parameters, and guide clinicians to best dose.
- Provide informed commentary on and interpretation of reported serum aminoglycoside concentrations and guide clinical management of such patients.
- Understand the potential pitfalls and problems with interpretation of reported aminoglycoside concentrations.

Rationale for therapeutic drug monitoring (TDM)

Aminoglycoside TDM is based on two facts. *Too much* aminoglycoside may cause patients harm, in terms of ototoxicity and nephrotoxicity. Ototoxicity, from uptake of drug into the cochlea and/or vestibular apparatus, may be difficult to detect unless severe and is generally irreversible or only partially reversible. Kidney damage from acute tubular necrosis is generally reversible on cessation of therapy. *Too little* aminoglycoside may harm by allowing the progress of overwhelming infection. Given the choice of death from infection, or hearing impairment, clinical microbiologists may mutter beneath their breath, '*Better a deaf patient, than a dead patient.*'

In summary, aminoglycoside TDM promotes targeted antimicrobial chemotherapy to improve outcomes and reduce potential toxicity.

Therapeutic range and evidence-base

Aminoglycosides are used to treat serious Gram-negative infections. The target range depends on putative organism/site of infection and dosing schedule employed: whether traditional, multiple-dose or extended-interval dosing. The therapeutic ranges for traditional aminoglycoside dosing are based largely on studies that demonstrated poor outcomes associated with suboptimal peak concentrations (Moore *et al.*, 1984).

By convention, for multiple-dose regimens, peak concentrations are drawn 1 h after intravenous bolus or intramuscular injection, and 30 min after a 30 min intravenous infusion. Trough concentrations are sampled immediately before the next dose is administered. Sample time, in relation to previous dosing, for both peak and trough concentrations, should be documented accurately to facilitate interpretation. (See Table 6.1.)

Higher peak concentrations, around 10–12 mg/L of gentamicin, are targeted for severe Gram-negative sepsis, while lower peak concentrations, around 3–6 mg/L, are acceptable for susceptible Gram-positive endocarditis, when used in synergy with beta-lactam antibiotics.

The target range for single daily, or extended-interval, dosing is generally a pre-dose trough concentration of less than 1 mg/L, or as determined by application of the Hartford nomogram (Nicolau *et al.*, 1995). Following administration of a fixed mg/kg dose, as a short infusion, a single serum concentration is drawn between 6 and 14 h after completion of administration. If the concentration is below the target, the dosage regimen is continued. If it is too high, the dosing interval is extended to allow a longer interval for elimination. Peak concentrations are not measured because it is assumed that with doses of 3–7 mg/kg/day, concentrations will be sufficiently high for bactericidal effect against most bacteria. The appropriateness of measuring pre-dose trough concentrations during extended-interval dosing has been questioned because

Table 6.1 Target range following multiple-dose therapy for aminoglycosides

Drug	Trough concentration (mg/L)	Peak concentration (mg/L)
Amikacin	<5	20–35
Gentamicin	<2	4–12
Netilmicin	<2	4–12
Tobramycin	<2	4–12

a measurable trough concentration may indicate overdose rather than correct dose (Begg *et al.*, 2001).

The rationale supporting higher-dose, extended-interval amino-glycoside regimens is based on the principle of concentration-dependent bacterial killing, the postantibiotic effect and the induction of adaptive resistance in Gram-negative bacteria (Barclay *et al.*, 1994). It is not appropriate, however, in all clinical cases and conventional, individu-alised therapy may be safer in endocarditis, pregnancy and renal impair-ment. Management of obese patients or those with altered hydrational states, such as those with marked ascites or pleural effusion or dehydra-tion, also presents a challenge in terms of what weight to use for dose calculation. In such cases, empirical dosing with measurement of peak and trough concentrations, and dose individualisation, may be more appropriate.

Once-daily, more accurately described as extended-interval, dosing aminoglycoside therapy has been adopted widely and with great enthu-siasm, though often guided by an equal measure of misunderstanding. The old adage 'If something is too good to be true, it probably is not true' has been used to describe once-daily aminoglycosides (Rotschafer and Ryback, 1994).

Best practice suggests that definition of a suitable target range for aminoglycoside therapy for individual patients should be discussed and agreed with a clinical microbiologist, who can give guidance on both likely organisms and susceptibility. A pharmacokineticist can then aim for the agreed target.

Pharmacokinetic profile (ADME)

Most aminoglycosides have low oral bioavailability (<1%) unless there is significant gastrointestinal inflammation. The bioavailability of neo-mycin is 3%.

Aminoglycosides predominantly distribute into body water, in par-ticular extracellular fluids. Distribution volume may be altered by any coexisting condition that affects fluid balance. Distribution volume will be greater in patients with ascites, oedema, pleural effusion, peritonitis, pregnancy, hypoalbuminaemia or AIDS or in the perioperative period. It is smaller in those who are dehydrated (Dager, 1994).

Aminoglycosides are eliminated mainly by glomerular filtration with some active secretion. Clearance approximates with creatinine clearance, which can be used for rough calculations.

Population data

Various volumes of distribution for aminoglycosides have been reported, from 0.06 to 0.84 L/kg, but account must be taken of any co-morbid state (Dager, 1994). Distribution volume is generally around 0.3 L/kg. A commonsense approach is to recognise interpatient variability and use:

$$V_d = 0.3 \, \text{L/kg} \pm 0.1$$

(Thummel and Shen, 2001). A patient with hypoalbuminaemia and ascites will have a volume tending towards 0.4 L/kg. A dehydrated individual will have a volume around 0.2 L/kg. To calculate a suitable dose of aminoglycoside, multiply the desired peak concentration by volume. Remember that the 1 h post-dose peak will be slightly less because there will be one hour's worth of elimination, but the method gives a good starting point for assessing appropriateness of a dose. If $V_d = 25 \, \text{L}$, and the desired peak is 8 mg/L, a dose of 8×25 or 200 mg should be given.

To predict V_d for those who are below ideal body weight, use actual weight. Remember that drug will not distribute into hypothetical body tissue. For patients who are obese, or 20% over ideal body weight, use dosing weight (Traynor *et al.*, 1995):

Dosing weight = Ideal body weight + (40% Excess body weight)

where

Excess body weight = (Total body weight − Ideal body weight)

This dosing weight recognises the fact that aminoglycoside distributes into fatty tissue, but to a lesser extent than in the rest of the body.

Equation resource – which equations to use and when

Only seven equations (6.1–6.7) are necessary in clinical practice for aminoglycoside interpretation.

$$k = \frac{\text{CL}}{V_d} \qquad (6.1)$$

where k = elimination rate constant, V_d = volume of distribution, and CL = aminoglycoside clearance. CL equates approximately with creatinine clearance. V_d can be approximated using 0.3 L/kg, which allows one to estimate a loading dose. An estimate can then be made of an individual's k value.

$$t_{1/2} = \frac{0.693}{k} \tag{6.2}$$

where $t_{1/2}$ = elimination half-life and k = elimination rate constant. A suitable dosing strategy can be calculated by dosing every 2, 3 or 4 half-lives, depending on what concentration decline is required between doses.

For peaks of 5 mg/L, and troughs around 1 mg/L, dose every 2 half-lives. The peak will fall from 5 mg/L to 2.5 mg/L in one $t_{1/2}$ and from 2.5 mg/L to 1.25 mg/L in another $t_{1/2}$. However, if you wish a peak of 12 mg/L and trough of 1 mg/L, a longer dosing interval is required. Concentrations will decline from 12 mg/L to 6 mg/L in one $t_{1/2}$, down to 3 mg/L in another $t_{1/2}$, then to 1.5 mg/L after another $t_{1/2}$, and down to 0.75 mg/L after a fourth interval of $t_{1/2}$. The dosing interval to achieve such a combination would thus be every 4 half-lives.

Note that the doses required in both cases above to produce a suitable concentration rise will be influenced by the V_d.

$$k = \frac{\ln C_{p1} - \ln C_{p2}}{\Delta t} \tag{6.3}$$

where k = elimination rate constant, C_{p1} = concentration at time 1, C_{p2} = concentration at time 2, and Δt = the time difference between samples drawn at time 1 and time 2. If two concentrations are sampled within the same dosing interval, after distribution is complete, an individualised patient-specific elimination rate constant can be calculated. If the concentration decline is less than 50%, accuracy decreases. To illustrate, consider the three cases in Box 6.1.

$$C_{p1} = \frac{D}{V_d} \exp(-k \, \Delta t) \tag{6.4}$$

This gives the concentration following a single intravenous bolus dose (D), where Δt is the time after injection.

Rearranging equation (6.4), V_d can be calculated thus:

$$V_d = \frac{D}{C_{p1}} \exp(-k \, \Delta t) \tag{6.5}$$

Box 6.1 The influence of sample time on precision of k and $t_{1/2}$. Three adults received a stat intravenous bolus dose of gentamicin, with two serum concentrations reported at different times

1. **Bill's 1 h post-dose concentration was 8 mg/L, and at 4 h was 6.8 mg/L.**

   $k = (\ln 8 - \ln 6.8)/3 = 0.05417\,h^{-1}$

   $t_{1/2} = 13\,h$

   If laboratory error was 5%, the concentrations could range over 8.4–7.6 mg/L and 7.1–6.5 mg/L.

   If concentration fell from 8.4 mg/L to 6.5 mg/L,

   $k = 0.08548\,h^{-1}$ $t_{1/2} = 8\,h$

   If concentration fell from 7.6 mg/L to 7.1 mg/L,

   $k = 0.02268\,h^{-1}$ $t_{1/2} = 31\,h$

2. **Bob's 1 h post-dose concentration was 8 mg/L, and at 13 h was 4.2 mg/L.**

   $k = (\ln 8 - \ln 4.2)/12 = 0.05370\,h^{-1}$

   $t_{1/2} = 13\,h$

   If laboratory error was 5%, the concentrations could range over 8.4–7.6 mg/L and 4.4–4 mg/L.

   If concentration fell from 8.4 mg/L to 4 mg/L,

   $k = 0.06183\,h^{-1}$ $t_{1/2} = 11\,h$

   If concentration fell from 7.6 mg/L to 4.4 mg/L,

   $k = 0.04555\,h^{-1}$ $t_{1/2} = 15\,h$

3. **Barry's 1 h post-dose concentration was 8 mg/L, and at 24 h was 2.3 mg/L.**

   $k = (\ln 8 - \ln 2.3)/23 = 0.05420\,h^{-1}$

   $t_{1/2} = 13\,h$

   If laboratory error was 5%, the concentrations could range over 8.4–7.6 mg/L and 2.4–2.2 mg/L.

   If concentration fell from 8.4 mg/L to 2.2 mg/L,

   $k = 0.05825\,h^{-1}$ $t_{1/2} = 12\,h$

   If concentration fell from 7.6 mg/L to 2.4 mg/L,

   $k = 0.05012\,h^{-1}$ $t_{1/2} = 14\,h$

   Precision is increased if concentrations are sampled at least one $t_{1/2}$ apart.

$$C_{p2} = C_{p1} \exp(-k \, \Delta t) \qquad\qquad (6.6)$$

C_{p2} = the concentration at any time Δt after some initial concentration C_{p1}.

$$C_{pt}^{ss} = \frac{D}{V_d} \frac{\exp(-kt)}{1 - \exp(-k\tau)} \qquad\qquad (6.7)$$

C_{pt}^{ss} = the steady-state concentration at time t following administration of a dose (D) of aminoglycoside, V_d = volume of distribution, k = elimination rate constant, and τ = dosing interval. Once a C_{p1h}^{ss} peak concentration is calculated, you can predict the trough from equation (6.6), where Δt is the time difference between the peak and trough; hence, 7 h if giving an 8-hourly schedule. Both calculations will give the same answer.

Reasons for request

A useful guiding principle for aminoglycoside concentration analysis is: 'Will it change how we manage the patient?' If a decision has been made to discontinue therapy the following day because of clinical improvement, measuring aminoglycoside concentrations today, 'Just to check,' is rather pointless. A cynic would suggest that we often measure concentrations simply because we can. It does not make such practice correct.

Better practice is to analyse concentrations at predetermined time points and make an informed interpretation about appropriateness, or otherwise, of dosing.

Generally, frequency of concentration analysis should be informed by the patient's clinical status, which changes with time. An otherwise healthy adult with normal renal function may not need to be monitored closely, and weekly trough concentration analysis will suffice if they are to receive an aminoglycoside for an extended time. Other patients require close monitoring, including the elderly, anephric patients, those with creatinine clearance less than 20 mL/min, those on dialysis, those taking concomitant ototoxic or nephrotoxic agents, patients with rapidly changing renal function, and patients in critical care. A critically ill, septic patient, with fluctuating renal function and changing fluid balance, should be monitored with daily concentration analysis and clinical pharmacokinetic interpretation.

Factors affecting therapeutic range including important drug interactions

Aminoglycosides are widely reported to interact with many diverse agents. Many interactions have an increased likelihood of nephrotoxicity when administered with concomitant nephrotoxins, such as vancomycin or loop diuretics. Few interactions appear to be mediated through a change in serum drug concentration. However, any drug that changes fluid balance could affect serum aminoglycoside concentrations. If a patient develops marked oedema, the concentration rise following a dose will decrease as volume increases. If they become dehydrated, the concentration rise will increase, because effectively their distribution volume decreases. This is more noticeable in the critical care setting where patient parameters can change acutely.

Clinical case studies

CASE STUDY 6.1

A.B., a 61-year-old woman, was admitted to hospital with chest infection. Her past medical history included bronchiectasis, chronic obstructive pulmonary disease, diabetes mellitus, hypertension, and recurrent pulmonary infection with Pseudomonas aeruginosa. Recent chest infections were treated with combinations of co-amoxiclav, ciprofloxacin, ceftazidime, colistin and Tazocin (piperacillin + tazobactam). She weighed 45.5 kg, height 160 cm (5 ft 3 in.). Her serum creatinine, which concurred with previous admissions, was 100 μmol/L.

Her drug history included oxitropium and Seretide (fluticasone + salmeterol) inhalers, nebulised salbutamol and ipratropium, enalapril, Human Mixtard 30 (biphasic human insulin) and an HRT patch.

In view of historical culture and sensitivity reports, A.B.'s symptoms were assumed to be an exacerbation of bronchiectasis, caused by Pseudomonas aeruginosa, and treatment with gentamicin and ceftazidime was recommended. A pharmacist was contacted on a Saturday afternoon for advice.

→

CASE STUDY 6.1 (continued)

From population estimates calculate A.B.'s pharmacokinetic parameters for gentamicin? What dose of gentamicin would you advise?

A.B. is underweight, hence for calculating pharmacokinetic parameters use her actual weight:

$$V_d = 0.3\,L/kg \times 45.5\,kg = 13.65\,L$$

$$\text{Creatinine clearance} = \frac{1.04 \times (140 - 61) \times 45.5}{100} = 37.4\,mL/min$$

Thus gentamicin clearance = 37.4 mL/min = 2.24 L/h.

$$k = CL/V_d = 0.16432\,h^{-1} \tag{6.8}$$

$$t_{1/2} = 4.2\,h \tag{6.9}$$

Using equation (6.4), if V_d equals 13.65 L, 140 mg of gentamicin should elevate the concentration at time zero by 10.3 mg/L, and at 1 h post dose by 8.7 mg/L.

A maintenance dose of 140 mg every 12 h should produce:

$$C_{1h}^{ss} = \frac{140}{13.65} \times \frac{e^{-0.16432 \times 1}}{1 - e^{-0.16432 \times 12}} = 10.1\,mg/L \tag{6.10}$$

$$C_{12h}^{ss} = \frac{140}{13.65} \times \frac{e^{-0.16432 \times 12}}{1 - e^{-0.16432 \times 12}} = 1.7\,mg/L \tag{6.11}$$

The pharmacist recommended a stat 140 mg dose by intravenous bolus injection, and that it should then be continued at 140 mg every 12 h.

The pharmacist also recommended monitoring pre- and post-dose concentrations around the afternoon dose on Sunday with clinical interpretation on Monday.

Concentrations sampled around the afternoon dose on Sunday, were reported on Monday as:

Pre-dose   1.3 mg/L
Post-dose   6 mg/L

What would you interpret from these trough and peak concentrations?

Peak and trough concentrations are not always what they appear and require careful interpretation (see Box 6.2, p. 125). The peak concentration is lower than expected. Possible explanations for a reduced peak include:

- Too low a dose
- Problems with sampling or administration: incomplete or late

$\rightarrow$

◑ CASE STUDY 6.1 (continued)

- Volume of distribution greater than population estimate

The trough concentration was also lower than predicted. Possible explanations for a low trough include:

- Elimination rate constant greater than population estimate
- Sample drawn late
- Previous dose given early

Note also that the concentration rise was 4.7 mg/L but was predicted as 8.6 mg/L.

Before making an interpretation one needs to exclude the possibilities outlined above. There was no obvious explanation for the disagreement between predicted and measured concentrations. What one can conclude, however, is that we need to extend the dosage interval, to allow elimination to less than 1 mg/L, before the next dose is given. A dose increase is also necessary, to produce a concentration rise of at least 7 or 8 mg/L. Calculation of V_d and k from a trough/peak pair such as this is difficult and necessitates many assumptions, which could not be confirmed with this limited data. A common-sense practical approach will suffice, however.

The pharmacist did both of the above and recommended a new dosage regimen of 220 mg IV bolus every 24 h.

When would you advise repeat concentrations be monitored?
It would be useful to measure concentrations at steady state to confirm the appropriateness or otherwise of the new dose. For a compromised patient, like A.B., whose pharmacokinetic parameters are different from the population values, with no clear reason why, the pharmacist advised staff to monitor pre- and post-dose concentrations around the morning dose on Tuesday with clinical interpretation the same day.

Concentrations, however, were requested around the evening dose on Tuesday. These were reported as:

Pre-dose   <1 mg/L
Post-dose   11.6 mg/L

Sputum from day 5 grew *Corynebacterium* species, which were sensitive to, and treated with, a 7-day course of oral co-amoxiclav. A.B. received 7 days of parenteral aminoglycoside therapy, and was discharged on day 15.

Box 6.2   Why are pre- and post-dose aminoglycoside concentrations so difficult to interpret?

We are reassured by aminoglycoside concentrations being within the target range. However, concentrations may be reported within range but the dose may still be inappropriate. What must we exclude before we can conclude appropriateness?

Pre-dose <1 mg/L: What does it mean?
- Dosing interval is acceptable.
- Or was the previous dose given early?
- Was the previous dose omitted and not given at all?
- Was an incomplete dose given previously?

Pre-dose >2 mg/L: What does it mean?
- Need to extend dosing interval.
- Or was the previous dose given late and thus not a true trough?
- Was the sample obtained early?
- Was it sampled from an administration line?

Post-dose peak within target range: What does it mean?
- Appropriate dose and frequency.
- Or was an incorrect dose administered?
- Was an incorrect sample time or method of administration used?
- Was a toxic dose sampled late?

Post-dose peak below target range: What does it mean?
- Dose too low.
- Or was the sample obtained late?
- Was an incomplete dose given previously?
- Was a dilute sample obtained?

Post-dose peak is above target range: What does it mean?
- Dose too high.
- Was the sample taken before complete distribution?
- Was the sample taken from an administration line?

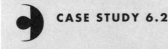

CASE STUDY 6.2

C.D. is a 19-year-old girl with cystic fibrosis. Her drug therapy includes pancreatic enzymes, prophylactic cefradine, vitamin supplements and
→

> **CASE STUDY 6.2** (continued)

ursodeoxycholic acid. She is colonised with Pseudomonas aeruginosa and receives intravenous antibiotics (tobramycin and cefazidime) every 3 months. Her weight is 55 kg, height 165 cm (5 ft 5 in.).
Biochemistry was normal with creatinine 67 μmol/L.

What target range would you suggest for tobramycin in C.D.?
Patients with cystic fibrosis have thick, tenacious sputum; hence, serum tobramycin concentrations should be targeted at peaks of 8–12 mg/L and trough concentrations less than 1 mg/L. Patients who are colonised with *Pseudomonas aeruginosa* also tend to receive large cumulative doses of aminoglycoside, from many repeat courses, and strict management of dosing is required to minimise the risk of toxicity.

From C.D.'s population parameters, estimate her distribution volume and tobramycin clearance? What dose would you recommend?

$$V_d = 0.3 \text{ L/kg} \times 55 \text{ kg} = 16.5 \text{ L}$$

Calculate C.D.'s creatinine clearance using the method of Cockcroft and Gault:

$$\text{Creatinine clearance} = \frac{1.04 \times (140 - 19) \times 55}{67} = 103.3 \text{ mL/min}$$

Thus tobramycin clearance = 6.2 L/h.

$$k = CL/V_d = 0.37576 \text{ h}^{-1} \tag{6.12}$$

$$t_{1/2} = 1.8 \text{ h} \tag{6.13}$$

Using equation (6.4), if V_d equals 16.5 L, a stat dose of 200 mg of tobramycin should elevate the concentration at time zero by 12.1 mg/L, and at 1 h post dose by 8.3 mg/L.
A maintenance dose of 200 mg every 8 h should produce:

$$C_{1h}^{ss} = \frac{200}{16.5} \times \frac{e^{-0.37576 \times 1}}{1 - e^{-0.37576 \times 8}} = 8.8 \text{ mg/L} \tag{6.14}$$

$$C_{8h}^{ss} = \frac{200}{16.5} \times \frac{e^{-0.37576 \times 8}}{1 - e^{-0.37576 \times 8}} = 0.6 \text{ mg/L} \tag{6.15}$$

C.D. does not wish to stay overnight for steady-state concentration analysis and does not want to keep coming back to hospital for bloods, so a stat dose is given with two timed concentrations sampled before next dose.

$\longrightarrow$

⬤ **CASE STUDY 6.2** (continued)

She received 240 mg of tobramycin by IV bolus injection at 1140 h. Concentrations were reported as:

1240 h, 1 h post   9.7 mg/L
1440 h, 3 h post   3.1 mg/L

What is C.D.'s actual tobramycin elimination rate constant and distribution volume?

$$k = \frac{\ln 9.7 - \ln 3.1}{2} = 0.57036 \text{ h}^{-1} \tag{6.16}$$

Note that in this case with k approaching 60%, accurate documentation of sample time is vital because a 10-min inaccuracy may significantly effect precision. Patients themselves are a useful, and underused, source of accurate information if they are asked beforehand to collect the time of administration and sampling.

$$t_{1/2} = 1.2 \text{ h} \tag{6.17}$$

$$V_d = \frac{240}{9.7} e^{-0.57036 \times 1} = 14 \text{ L} \tag{6.18}$$

Population parameters are similar to individualised values, so the results seem plausible.

The advantage of sampling two timed concentrations, following a stat dose, is that an individual's pharmacokinetic parameters can be calculated and therapy individualised from the beginning, rather than after three or four doses.

What dose would you recommend now?
Using these figures and a dose of tobramycin of 240 mg every 8 h, the predicted steady-state concentrations are:

$$C_{1h}^{ss} = \frac{240}{14} \times \frac{e^{-0.57036 \times 1}}{1 - e^{-0.57036 \times 8}} = 9.8 \text{ mg/L} \tag{6.19}$$

$$C_{8h}^{ss} = \frac{240}{14} \times \frac{e^{-0.57036 \times 8}}{1 - e^{-0.57036 \times 8}} = 0.2 \text{ mg/L} \tag{6.20}$$

When would you advise repeat concentrations be monitored?
As k is approaching 60%, one can be fairly confident that tobramycin will be adequately cleared between dosing within an 8-hourly dosing schedule. We also have proof that a dose of 240 mg will elevate the concentration by 9.7 mg/L. Treatment is for 2 weeks. A trough concentration after a week of treatment would be useful to assess clearance and highlight whether any

$\rightarrow$

CASE STUDY 6.2 (continued)

third-compartment accumulation was taking place. A young, fit, healthy teenager like C.D., however, does not require intensive concentration analysis following the initial concentration analysis.

CASE STUDY 6.3

F.G., a 45-year-old male with acute myeloid leukaemia became pyrexial a week after completing his second course of chemotherapy (daunorubicin and cytarabine). Antibiotic therapy was commenced with intravenous ceftazidime and vancomycin through a Hickman catheter, pending culture and sensitivity results. Treatment was continued for 5 days, although the blood culture results were inconclusive and the patient remained pyrexial. C-reactive protein was elevated at 108 mg/L.

Biochemical parameters were within normal limits, and haematology results were deranged: urea 4.7 mmol/L, creatinine 73 μmol/L, WBC 0.2 × 10⁹/L, haemoglobin 8 g/dL, platelets 2 × 10⁹/L, neutrophils 0.1 × 10⁹/L. F.G.'s weight was 102 kg, height 167.6 cm (5 ft 6 in.).

On day 5 following discussion with clinical microbiology, therapy was changed to intravenous Tazocin (piperacillin + tazobactam) 4.5 g every 8 h and gentamicin as a single daily dose.

Is single-daily dosing appropriate for this patient?
Single-daily, or extended interval, dosing of aminoglycoside is appropriate for certain infections in those with normal renal function. For patients who are obese, use ideal body weight to calculate creatinine clearance:

$$\text{Creatinine clearance} = \frac{1.23 \times (140 - 145) \times 63.8}{73} = 102 \text{ mL/min}$$

F.G. has normal renal function, therefore a fixed mg/kg daily dose of gentamicin would be appropriate. The initial dosing interval should be based on an estimate of renal function: if creatinine clearance is 60 mL/min or more, dose every 24 h; if it is 59–40 mL/min, dose every 36 h; and if it is 39–20 mL/min, dose every 48 h. Subsequent interval adjustments are made in accord with the Hartford nomogram (Nicolau *et al.*,1995).

What weight should be used to calculate his dose? What dose would you recommend? How should it be administered?
F.G. is obese. His actual weight is 102 kg. His ideal body weight is 63.8 kg.

→

◗ **CASE STUDY 6.3** (continued)

For obese patients, doses should be calculated using dosing weight (Traynor *et al.*,1995):

$$\text{Excess body weight} = (\text{Total body weight} - \text{Ideal body weight})$$
$$= 102 - 63.8 = 38.2\,\text{kg}$$
$$\text{Dosing weight} = \text{Ideal body weight} + (40\%\ \text{Excess body weight})$$
$$= 63.8 + (40\% \times 38.2)$$
$$= 79.1\,\text{kg}$$

Dosing weight recognises that aminoglycoside distributes into fatty tissue, but to a lesser extent than the rest of the body, and is appropriate for single-daily dosing (Nicolau *et al.*, 1995).

A dose of 7 mg/kg dosing weight, or 554 mg, would be appropriate. Gentamicin is available as a 40 mg/mL solution, so round the dose to the nearest 40 mg to make the dose volume sensible. In this case the patient could have 560 mg or 520 mg in 50 mL of sodium chloride 0.9% injection, infused over 60 min.

When would you advise measuring concentrations?
There is no point measuring the peak concentration after such a large single dose because it will be above 20 mg/L, which is sufficiently high for bactericidal effect against most bacteria. The method commonly used in practice is to measure a single serum concentration drawn between 6 and 14 h after completion of administration, and to compare the result with the Hartford nomogram (Nicolau *et al.*, 1995).

F.G. received a dose of 560 mg gentamicin in 50 mL of sodium chloride 0.9% injection, infused over 60 min. The concentration, reported 9 h after complete administration, was 1.4 mg/L.

What would you interpret from this?
The reported concentration lies below the dosing interval line. The line indicates whether the dose interval should be 24-, 36- or 48-hourly. If it is close to or above the line, the dosing interval should be extended to avoid accumulation and provide an appropriate drug-free period. If it is below the line, continue with the same interval. The interpretation would thus be to continue therapy with 560 mg every 24 h if there was an appropriate clinical response.

F.G. had good clinical response, was apyrexial and completed a 6-day course of gentamicin and Tazocin. His renal function and fluid balance remained stable throughout and further gentamicin concentration measurements were thought unnecessary.

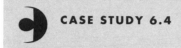

CASE STUDY 6.4

G.H., a 66-year-old man, was admitted to ITU following cardiac arrest and repair of a ruptured aortic aneurysm. His past medical history included chronic obstructive pulmonary disease and ischaemic heart disease. He was a smoker. His drug history comprised prophylactic aspirin, plus beclometasone and salbutamol inhalers. His weight was around 80 kg.

On day 16, MRSA and Pseudomonas aeruginosa were isolated from sputum and treatment commenced with teicoplanin and ciprofloxacin. On day 20, microbiology reported the latest sputum to contain a species of Pseudomonas aeruginosa that was resistant to ciprofloxacin. He was commenced on gentamicin and ciprofloxacin was discontinued.

Other treatment included noradrenaline (norepinephrine) infusion; teicoplanin 400 mg daily; intravenous ranitidine 50 mg t.d.s.; subcutaneous enoxaparin and nebulised salbutamol and ipratropium.

The on-call pharmacist was contacted at 1900 h and asked, 'What dose of gentamicin should we give?'

What dose would you recommend?
Population pharmacokinetic parameters in the critical care setting are notoriously problematic. Haemodynamic changes happen acutely and prediction at one time point may not accurately represent future status. Rather than hypothesising, the author would suggest, administer a reasonable dose and measure the individual's pharmacokinetic response. As the patient weighed around 80 kg, the pharmacist recommended: 240 mg stat to effect a concentration around 10 mg/L, sample two timed concentrations, store in the fridge overnight, and analyse first thing in the morning.

A stat dose of 240 mg of IV gentamicin was administered at 2030 h on day 20. Concentrations were reported the following day as:

2130 h   4.5 mg/L
0400 h   1.2 mg/L

What is G.H.'s actual elimination rate constant and volume of distribution? How likely are these results?
From the reported concentrations, an individualised pharmacokinetic profile was calculated as:

$$k = \frac{\ln 4.5 - \ln 1.2}{6.5} = 0.20335 \ h^{-1} \tag{6.21}$$

$$t_{1/2} = 3.4 \ h \tag{6.22}$$

$\rightarrow$

● **CASE STUDY 6.4** (continued)

$$V_d = \frac{240}{4.5} = e^{-0.20335 \times 1} = 43.5\,L \tag{6.23}$$

This equates with a volume of 0.54 L/kg.

The population estimate of volume of distribution, assuming an ideal body weight of around 80 kg, is

$$V_d = 0.3\,L/kg \times 80\,kg = 24\,L$$

Is the patient likely to have a volume of distribution that is almost double the expected population value?

Remember that population estimates of distribution volume are drawn from small studies that may not reflect the individual patient under consideration. In general terms, the distribution volume of gentamicin in adult patient's ranges from 0.2 to 0.4 L/kg. These figures, however, do not reflect the extreme circumstances within the ITU or HDU, where fluid overload, hypoalbuminaemia, septic shock, long-term mechanical ventilation, pleural effusion and ascites, among others, will influence distribution. Two reports detail the volume of distribution as mean and range, in surgical ITUs, as 0.29, 0.11–0.54 L/kg (Mann *et al.*, 1987) and 0.20, 0.06–0.63 L/kg (Zaske *et al.*, 1980). The predicted volume of 0.54 L/kg is thus by no means impossible. These figures do not, however, confirm probability.

G.H., was very oedematous with fluid overload. He was commenced on furosemide.

What other explanations are there for the small concentration rise, which was interpreted as a large distribution volume?

- Incomplete dose administration. It was assumed that 240 mg distributed in the body to achieve a concentration of 4.5 mg/L. What if only 120 mg was given, or 140 mg was given and 100 mg was 'lost' or spilt during administration?
- Was the sample drawn 60 min after complete administration? How was the gentamicin given? Was it by a slow IV infusion, or by IV bolus injection? At this point it was unclear how the drug was administered.
- Was the blood sample contaminated with a saline lock or heparinised saline?

If there is great variation in distribution volume when the individualised estimate is compared with population estimates, try to find an explanation.

→

> **CASE STUDY 6.4** (continued)

What target concentration range should we aim for in a patient like this?
In a case with positive blood cultures it is always worth discussing with a clinical microbiologist and agreeing a suitable target concentration. In this patient the target set was a peak of about 10 mg/L and trough less than 2 mg/L.

What dose would you recommend to achieve a peak of about 10 mg/L and trough of less than 2 mg/L?
Using these individualised parameters, the pharmacist predicted the steady-state peak and trough that would result from a dose of 320 mg every 12 h:

$$C_{1h}^{ss} = \frac{320}{43.5} \times \frac{e^{-0.20335 \times 1}}{1 - e^{-0.20335 \times 12}} = 6.6 \text{ mg/L} \tag{6.24}$$

$$C_{12h}^{ss} = \frac{320}{43.5} \times \frac{e^{-0.20335 \times 12}}{1 - e^{-0.20335 \times 12}} = 0.7 \text{ mg/L} \tag{6.25}$$

The pharmacist recommended a dose of 320 mg twice daily. If the parameters were true, this would not achieve a peak of 10 mg/L, but there was question as to the validity of the calculated V_d. A caveat was placed that the patient could probably tolerate a greater dose but their clinical condition might change quite quickly. Pre- and post-dose concentrations were recommended the following day, to prove or disprove adequacy of the new dosing regimen.

Charts suggested a negative fluid balance of 300 mL on day 21 and a negative balance of 3000 mL on day 22. Concentrations were reported on day 23 as:

Pre-dose   2.3 mg/L
Post-dose   8.9 mg/L

What additional information do you require before interpreting these concentrations?
Before interpreting any concentration you must check the *exact dosing history* and *method of administration*, and *site* and *time* of any *blood samples*. This is especially critical in the ITU setting. Without this information, any subsequent interpretation will be difficult.

On further investigation it transpired that the gentamicin was administered in 100 mL of sodium chloride 0.9% over approximately 10 min, but possibly longer. Concentration was sampled 1 h after the infusion started, or possibly stopped, but it did vary and was not consistent. Any subsequent interpretation in a case like this must be dubious, depending on what assumptions have been made.

The pharmacist noted 'Large diuresis with furosemide so V_d decreased. This could give a peak of up to 12 mg/L but $t_{1/2} = 6$ h so will clear it. Asked for

$\longrightarrow$

> **CASE STUDY 6.4** (continued)

pre on Sunday if possible or pre/post Monday morning as diuresis likely to continue.' The pharmacokinetic recommendation for gentamicin was for 360 mg once daily, at 1000 h, with omission of the evening dose.

The dose of gentamicin prescribed by the clinician, however, was 320 mg once daily. G.H. received a dose on day 24 and concentrations were sampled on day 25. These were reported as:

Pre-dose concentration	<1 mg/L
Post-dose concentration	14.2 mg/L

What interpretation would you draw from the reported concentrations and what dose would you recommend now?

Note that the concentration rise is 13 or 14 mg/L following a dose of 320 mg. Previously 320 mg produced a concentration rise of 6.6 mg/L and 240 mg produced a rise of 4.5 mg/L following the first dose. These results are not proportional:

- Has there been a tremendous change in distribution volume? Does this reflect changing fluid balance within G.H.?
- Have different methods or processes of drug administration been used? Were the doses all given by IV bolus injection, or were some given by pulsed infusion over variable times?
- Were the sample times different in relation to drug administration? Were the post-dose concentrations drawn at the same time after drug administration or were they sampled during distribution phase or 60 min after commencing drug administration rather than completion?

When interpreting pre-dose and post-dose concentration pairs, it is useful to consider concentration rise and how plausible the concentrations are when compared with previous results.

Following these results, the pharmacist recommended, by proportion, a dose decrease to 280 mg once daily. Concentrations sampled on day 28 were reported as:

Pre-dose concentration	<1 mg/L
Post-dose concentration	10.8 mg/L
6 h post-dose concentration	3.6 mg/L

What are G.H.'s actual elimination rate constant and half-life? How appropriate is the current dose?

From these figures an individualised k can be calculated thus:

$$k = \frac{\ln 10.8 - \ln 3.6}{5} = 0.21972 \text{ h}^{-1} \qquad (6.26)$$

$\rightarrow$

> **CASE STUDY 6.4** (continued)

$$t_{1/2} = 3.2\,h \tag{6.27}$$

With a $t_{1/2}$ of 3.2 h, a dosing interval of 12 h would allow the concentration to decline to around 10% between doses (50%→25%→12.5% plus). The dose was appropriate as the concentration rise was measured as greater than 9.8 mg/L. Hence a new dosage regimen of 280 mg 12-hourly was recommended.

The patient was scheduled to receive only one more day of gentamicin, so no further dose adjustment was advised.

References/Further reading

Barclay M L, Begg E J, Hickling K G (1994). What is the evidence for once-daily aminoglycoside therapy? *Clin Pharmacokinet* 27: 32–48.

Begg E J, Barclay M L, Kirkpatrick C M J (2001). The therapeutic monitoring of antimicrobial agents. *Br J Clin Pharmacol* 52: 35S–45S.

Dager W E (1994). Aminoglycoside pharmacokinetics: volume of distribution in specific adult patient subgroups. *Ann Pharmacother* 28: 944–951.

Mann H J, Fuhs D N, Awang R, Ndemo F A, Cerra F B (1987). Altered aminoglycoside pharmacokinetics in critically ill patients with sepsis. *Clin Pharm* 6: 148–153.

Moore R D, Smith C R, Lietman P S (1984). The association of aminoglycoside plasma levels with mortality in patients with gram-negative bacteremia. *J Infect Dis* 149: 443–448.

Nicolau D P, Freeman C D, Belliveau P P, Nightingale C H, Ross J W, Quintiliani R (1995). Experience with a once-daily aminoglycoside program administered to 2,184 adult patients. *Antimicrob Agents Chemother* 39: 650–655.

Rotschafer J C, Rybak M J (1994). Single daily dosing of aminoglycosides: a commentary. *Ann Pharmacother* 28: 797–801.

Thummel K E, Shen D D (2001). Appendix 2. Design and optimization of dosage regimens: Pharmacokinetic data. In: Hardman J G, Limbird L E, Goodman L S and Gilman A, eds. *Goodman and Gilman's The Pharmacological Basis of Therapeutics*, 10th edn. New York: McGraw-Hill, 1963.

Traynor A M, Nafziger A N, Bertino J S (1995). Aminoglycoside dosing weight correction factors for patients of various body sizes. *Antimicrob Agents Chemother* 39: 545–548.

Zaske D E, Cipolle R J, Strate R J (1980). Gentamicin dosage requirements: wide interpatient variations in 242 surgery patients with normal renal function. *Surgery* 87: 164–169.

7

Digoxin

Graham Mould

Aims and learning outcomes

After completing this chapter, readers will be able to:

- Discuss the rationale for digoxin therapeutic drug monitoring (TDM).
- Describe the factors that affect the interpretation of digoxin concentrations.
- Design suitable dosing regimens for digoxin using population data and patient biochemical and physical parameters.
- Solve practical pharmacokinetic problems based on digoxin therapy.

Rationale for therapeutic drug monitoring (TDM)

Patient compliance

Many patients are erratic in their compliance. In particular, when patients arrive in hospital, medication is given on a regular basis. In order to ascertain compliance beforehand, it may be prudent for an initial sample to be taken for drug measurement.

It is worth noting that undetected concentrations may correspond to the lower limit of sensitivity of the assay. In these cases an estimate may be useful.

Multiple drug therapy

Drug interactions (see later) are an important indicator for drug measurement. In a recent study evaluating over 600 patients, the authors found increases in digoxin concentrations of between 20% and 60% in patients receiving P-glycoprotein inhibitors (such as amiodarone, ciclosporin, quinidine and verapamil) in a hospital in Sweden (Englund *et al.*, 2004).

Confirming drug toxicity

While the signs of digoxin toxicity, such as nausea, vomiting, abdominal pain and arrhythmias, are well recognised, it is useful to confirm toxicity with a serum measurement. The value may be useful for determining the length of time required for the concentration to reach therapeutic concentrations.

Altered disease states

Since digoxin is almost exclusively eliminated renally, any deteriorating renal function will require digoxin monitoring. Digoxin toxicity is increased in cases of hypokalaemia and hypercalcaemia. Hyperthyroidism makes patients more resistant to digoxin, whereas patients who are hypothyroid require lower doses.

Inadequate therapeutic response

If there is a poor response to digoxin, even with recommended doses, then a digoxin measurement is useful to determine whether there is an adequate amount present.

Relationship between serum concentration and response

Clinical response

Smith (1973) reported that the extent of Na^+, K^+-ATPase inhibition by digoxin is related to the serum concentration, and that this is related to increasing dosage. Further clinical studies by Hoeschen and Cuddy (1975) showed that serum digoxin concentration bore a close relationship to the myocardial effects by demonstrating that changes in left ventricular ejection volume correlated reasonably well with steady-state serum digoxin concentration. These patients were in cardiac failure; using patients in atrial fibrillation, other workers (Redfors, 1972; Aronson et al., 1977) have found good correlations between serum concentration and the slowing of ventricular rate.

Although the serum digoxin concentration has not conclusively been shown to be correlated with the various clinical effects of digoxin, most workers prefer to maintain the steady-state concentration between 1.0 and 2.0 ng/mL (1.3–2.6 nmol/L). Furthermore, a number of studies have demonstrated that there is a significant difference between the mean values of digoxin concentrations with and without toxicity, but that there is a variable overlap (Aronson *et al.*, 1978). Nevertheless, the positive inotropic effect begins at low concentrations, and increases as serum concentration increases. The usual range for the inotropic effect is 1.0–1.5 ng/mL, whereas chronotropic effects are seen at concentrations greater than 1.5 ng/mL. Some patients, especially young children and neonates, will tolerate higher concentrations and may require up to 2.5 ng/mL or even higher. A subgroup analysis of the Digitalis Investigation Group trial suggested that the effectiveness of digoxin in men with heart failure and a left ejection fraction of 45% or less may be optimised in the range 0.5–0.8 ng/mL (Li Wan Po *et al.*, 2003).

In general, there is therefore a reasonable relationship between digoxin serum concentration and its therapeutic effect. Toxicity may start to be observed at concentrations above 1.5 ng/mL, although toxicity is virtually certain above 3.0 ng/mL (Aronson *et al.*, 1978).

Pharmacokinetic profile (ADME)

Absorption

The bioavailability (*F*) of digoxin is variable. For tablets, it has been suggested to be 0.70 with a range of 0.55–0.78 (Sheiner *et al.*, 1981). However, the figure of 0.63 is the one normally used. Surgical interventions in the gastrointestinal tract appear to have little effect on digoxin absorption. Intramuscular digoxin is painful and causes muscle necrosis, and this route should be avoided if possible. The *F* factor appeared to be 0.82 when calculated in a study using eight subjects (Greenblatt *et al.*, 1973). The salt factor (*S*) for digoxin is 1.0.

The absorption half-life as determined in fasting subjects is 27.1 ± 6.8 min (Lloyd *et al.*, 1978). This indicates that absorption is rapid, with peak concentrations in the central compartment at 1 h or so post dose. These high initial concentrations in blood do not necessarily result in cardiac toxicity, although some of the peripheral effects may be seen. Digoxin cardiac toxicity is more related to tissue concentrations of digoxin, and hence the post-distribution phase.

Distribution

Digoxin pharmacokinetics is described by a two-compartment model. The heart behaves as though it is in the second, or tissue, compartment.

The concentration of digoxin differs throughout the body, the highest being in the myocardium. In a post-mortem study, Doherty *et al.*, using tritiated digoxin, found a relatively constant ratio of myocardium to serum concentration of about 30 : 1. However, in a later study using papillary muscle taken from patients undergoing heart surgery, Hartel *et al.* (1976) found that the ratio of myocardial tissue to serum digoxin concentrations was 67 : 1. Protein binding is low and of the order of 26% (Ohnhaus *et al.*, 1972).

The distribution phase is usually complete by 6–8 h after an oral dose. It is only during the beta or elimination phase that digoxin is in equilibrium between serum and tissue. Accordingly, for the serum concentration to best reflect cardiac activity and clearance, it is important that samples should be drawn during the beta phase. Samples must therefore be taken at least 6 h after an oral dose or 4 h after IV dosing. The ideal time is probably 11 h after an oral dose (Nicholson *et al.*, 1980), but this timing may not be practical, especially if the dose is taken in the morning. Traditionally, 6 h remains the most frequently quoted time of sampling.

The apparent volume of distribution (V_d) has been reported to be about 476 L (Jusko *et al.*, 1974), although a larger figure of 8.5 ± 3.5 L/kg was suggested by Sheiner *et al.* (1981) when reviewing the literature at that time. Other workers use 7.3 L/kg, although for the old and frail one should use 6 L/kg. The V_d is this large because of extensive binding to skeletal muscle and myocardial tissue. Digoxin distributes poorly into adipose tissue (Ewy *et al.*, 1971); ideal body weight (see Chapter 3) is therefore a better estimate of V_d. Volume of distribution is reduced in cardiac failure and advanced renal failure, and values of 3 L/kg and below have been observed (Aronson and Grahame-Smith, 1976), although the average value has been quoted to be 4.2 ± 1.6 L/kg.

Elimination

Digoxin is eliminated largely by renal excretion. Most of the drug in urine is recoverable as unchanged drug. A small amount is metabolised by gut bacteria prior to absorption. However, in a small proportion of individuals (about 10%) this metabolism is increased, so that approximately 30–40% of the digoxin in urine consists of the so-called 'reduction products'.

It is known that the clearance is very dependent on kidney function and notice should always be taken of deteriorating creatinine clearance, and the digoxin clearance should be assessed. The half-life of digoxin in patients with normal renal function is about 40 h. This can be substantially increased in the face of reduced kidney function.

Population data

Bioavailability

F (oral tablets) = 0.63 (N.B. other figures have been used,
e.g. 0.70.)

F (oral elixir) = 0.75

Distribution

There are two methods for estimating V_d from population data, namely:

$$V_d = 3.12CL_{cr} + 3.84IBW$$

where CL_{cr} is creatinine clearance in mL/min (Sheiner et al., 1977) and IBW is ideal body weight (see Chapter 3); or

$$V_d = 7.3 \text{ L/kg} \qquad (6 \text{ L/kg in elderly frail patients})$$

Clearance

The renal clearance is approximately equal to the creatinine clearance:

$$CL_{total} = CL_{metabolic} + CL_{renal}$$

The calculated clearance has been reported by various authors (Koup et al., 1975; Dobbs et al., 1976; Sheiner et al., 1977). The most widely used is that of Sheiner et al. (1977), who measured serum digoxin at steady state in two groups of patients. One group was 99 inpatients with a degree of cardiac failure and impaired renal function. The other group was 42 outpatients. Regression equations were obtained and, when transposed from surface area to body weight, the relationships were as follows. With some degree of heart failure:

$$CL \text{ (L/h)} = 0.053CL_{cr} + 0.02IBW$$

Without heart failure:

$$CL \text{ (L/h)} = 0.06CL_{cr} + 0.05IBW$$

A recent study of the kinetics in 51 paediatric patients with an age range of 6 days to 1 year calculated the digoxin clearance to achieve a steady-state digoxin concentration of 1.5 ng/mL to be

$$CL \text{ (L/h/kg)} = 0.237[1 + 0.094 + \text{Age (months)}]$$

Equation resource

Volume of distribution

An additional method of calculating the volume is from Jusko *et al.* (1974), who defined V_d as a function of creatinine clearance using a Michaelis–Menten type equation. Thus,

$$V_d = V_a + \frac{V_n \times CL_{cr}}{K_d + CL_{cr}}$$

where $V_a = 226\,L/1.73\,m^2$; $V_n = 298\,L/1.73\,m^2$; $K_d = 29.1\,mL/min/1.73\,m^2$; $CL_{cr} = mL/min/1.73\,m^2$. ($V_a$ is the minimum digoxin distribution volume to be expected in a severely uraemic patient; V_n and K_d are Michaelis–Menten constants producing a maximum V_d value approaching $V_a + V_n$ in patients with normal renal function; CL_{cr} is the calculated creatinine clearance (see Case study 7.1).)

These workers found a better correlation using this formula, rather than 510 L, for the volume of distribution in patients with creatinine clearances less than 25 mL/min. From a consideration of the above formulae for V_d, 7.3 L/kg should be used when no creatinine clearance is available, and the Sheiner formula when creatinine clearance is known, even when there is impaired renal function. In the latter case, the Jusko formula might be equally appropriate.

When the weight of the patient is being considered, IBW should be used if the patient is greater than 20% obese. If actual body weight is less than IBW, then actual body weight (ABW) is used.

Clearance

In practice, the values obtained from these calculations may overestimate clearance, especially for elderly patients without heart failure. Creatinine clearance is in mL/min, weight is in kg and IBW should be used if obesity is greater than 20%.

Reasons for request

There are controversies regarding the usefulness of drug measurement in general and for digoxin in particular. However, experience has taught that digoxin is a useful drug to measure, when used correctly (Vozeh, 1987). The therapeutic range has been quoted as 1.0–2.0 ng/mL, which in SI units is 1.3–2.6 nmol/L, although some centres use 0.9–2.6 nmol/L.

The following are indications for measurement of digoxin concentrations.

Suspected subtherapeutic concentrations

These may occur because of no observed improvement or worsening of heart failure or atrial fibrillation at a dose calculated to be sufficient for therapeutic maintenance.

Suspected noncompliance

Noncompliance is a problem especially in the elderly, and therapeutic drug monitoring is useful in these circumstances. This may present an additional problem on hospital admission, which may necessitate a random sample being taken.

Suspected supratherapeutic concentrations

Supratherapeutic levels may be detected by clinical side-effects such as unusual fatigue, anorexia, nausea or vomiting. Cardiac side-effects, which may be difficult to distinguish from the underlying disease itself, mainly consist of ventricular arrhythmias, which may be characterised by ECG recordings. The most common arrhythmias are premature ventricular complexes (ectopic beats) including bigeminy, AV junctional escape beats or tachycardia, second- or third-degree heart block, atrial tachycardia with block and ventricular tachycardia. In these cases, immediate action should be taken and the dose should be stopped or reduced. A blood sample taken at this time for a digoxin measurement will confirm the diagnosis of digoxin toxicity and will be helpful in deciding future therapy by calculation of suitable alternative dose regimens or prediction of the time taken for drug to be eliminated. Again, in exceptional cases a random sample may give useful information.

Changing renal or thyroid function

When renal function is deteriorating as measured by a rising serum creatinine, digoxin measurement is worthwhile. Changing thyroid function may be another reason for monitoring digoxin.

The addition of other medication

The addition of amiodarone, quinidine or high doses of verapamil to the drug regimen should be carefully monitored.

Factors altering therapeutic range

A number of factors should be taken into account when assessing a digoxin concentration. The most important consideration is that hypokalaemia (as well as hypomagnesaemia and hypercalcaemia) increase myocardial sensitivity to digoxin. Many diuretics do cause low potassium (indapamide in particular), and when the potassium is less than 3 mmol/L toxicity any digoxin concentration may cause toxicity. Other factors include severe coronary arterial disease or a previous myocardial infarction, which may predispose to digoxin toxicity.

Goldman *et al.* (1975) reported that patients with stable, chronic atrial fibrillation were well controlled with levels less than 2.0 ng/mL (2.6 nmol/L). Those not controlled had acute or chronic atrial fibrillation with unstable conditions such as postoperative state, sepsis, or pulmonary embolism. This latter group often required concentrations above 2.0 ng/mL for control, with no signs of toxicity.

A number of drugs will alter the disposition of digoxin and when added to the therapy may affect the blood level observed (for review see Rodin and Johnson, 1988).

Drugs that will reduce digoxin absorption

Concurrent administration of liquid *aluminium or magnesium hydroxide*, or *kaolin and pectin* mixtures may reduce digoxin absorption. *Colestyramine* interferes with digoxin absorption and *colestipol* is known to bind to digoxin and has been shown to reduce its half-life in patients receiving colestipol every 6 h. *Neomycin* and *bran fibre* have also been shown to reduce digoxin absorption.

Drugs that will increase bioavailability

Some antibiotics are known to inhibit bacterial degradation in the gut to inactive metabolites in those patients who metabolise digoxin. *Erythromycin* has been reported to increase digoxin concentrations in about 10% of patients (Maxwell *et al.*, 1989). This effect may be evident for up to 2 weeks after stopping antibiotic therapy. A similar effect has been reported with clarithromycin (Rengelshausen *et al.*, 2003).

Interactions with antiarrhythmic drugs

Most patients exhibit a 2-fold to 3-fold rise in serum concentration following *quinidine* and digoxin. A decrease in the apparent digoxin V_d by

10–35% and a decreased rate of elimination are the accepted mechanisms. The result is a decrease in digoxin clearance of between 36% and 64% (Williams *et al.*, 1992). Digoxin and *amiodarone* is another well-documented interaction, which appears to be of greater magnitude in children than in adults. A reduction in both the renal and nonrenal digoxin clearance and an increase in digoxin bioavailability are the most likely explanations. *Verapamil* (>160 mg/day) decreases the total digoxin clearance by up to 30%. This effect may vary with time. Contradictory results have been reported of the interaction between digoxin and *diltiazem* and *nifedipine*. It is clear that whenever other antiarrhythmic drugs are added to digoxin therapy, caution needs to be exercised.

Interactions with diuretics

Furosemide, by virtue of its hypokalaemic effect, may decrease the renal tubular excretion of digoxin. *Spironolactone* may also inhibit the renal clearance of digoxin, giving rise to elevated concentrations. In addition, spironolactone and its metabolites have been shown to interfere with some of the digoxin assay methods, although the interference is small (Pleasants *et al.*, 1989).

Miscellaneous pharmacokinetic interactions

Some of the nonsteroidal anti-inflammatory drugs (NSAIDs) have been shown to increase digoxin levels, e.g. *indometacin* and *ibuprofen*. The evidence for interactions with other NSAIDs is not convincing.

Cardiac failure

Congestive heart failure may lead to a decrease in renal function, which will decrease the elimination of digoxin. In severe failure, there may also be an increased volume of distribution due to oedema. When this occurs, lower levels will result, although Ohnhaus *et al.* (1979) reported no change in digoxin kinetics in patients with severe right-sided heart failure.

Analytical methodology

A number of methods are available for digoxin analysis. Radioimmunoassay (RIA) is the most acceptable, although recent fluorescence polarisation immunoassay (FPIA) reagents have resulted in the increasing use of this method, e.g. by the Abbott TDX. The major disadvantage of the latter method is the requirement for a prior centrifugation step. Often these assays have detected metabolites and endogenous digoxin-like immunoreactive substance (DLIS), a compound that has been detected in the plasma of neonates not treated with the drug. Furthermore, patients with renal dysfunction, hepatic disease, hypertension and pregnancy also may have measurable DLIS (Stone *et al.*, 1990). The interference is probably more prevalent with RIA than with FPIA.

Other potential interfering agents include the antidote to acute digoxin poisoning, namely Digibind (Wells *et al.*, 1992). It should only be used when a significant overdose has been taken, such as through incorrect dosing. Digoxin concentrations should be measured prior to giving Digibind since, following its administration, blood measurements are of no use because of extensive interference.

Patients receiving digitoxin or other cardiac glycosides (e.g. digitalis leaf) will also produce erroneous results.

Clinical case study

CASE STUDY 7.1

A woman of weight 65 kg and height 160 cm (5 ft 3 in.) and who is 50 years old is in acute atrial fibrillation (AF). Her serum creatinine is 180 µmol/L.

Calculate an IV loading dose and oral maintenance dose
(1)   Calculate obesity:

$$IBW \text{ (female)} = 45.5 \text{ kg} + 2.3 \text{ (every inch above 5 feet)}$$
$$IBW = 52.4 \text{ kg}$$
$$\text{Obesity \%} = [(65 - 52.4) \times 100]/52.4 = 25\%$$

Therefore, IBW should be used as the obesity factor is greater than 20%.
(2)   Calculate creatinine clearance CL_{cr}:

$$CL_{cr} = \frac{1.04 \times (140 - Age) \times IBW}{Serum\ creatinine}$$
$$CL_{cr} = 27.0 \text{ mL/min}$$

$\rightarrow$

(3) Calculate volume of distribution V_d using the formula for renal impairment:

$$V_d = 3.12CL_{cr} + 3.84(IBW)$$
$$= 3.12(27) + 3.84(52)$$
$$V_d = 284\,L$$

(4) Calculate loading dose LD (aim for C_p of 1.5 µg/L):

$$LD = \frac{V_d \times C_p}{S \times F}$$
$$= \frac{284 \times 1.5}{1.0 \times 1.0}$$
$$LD = 426\,\mu g$$

Therefore, a loading dose of 500 µg IV may be given. This would achieve a concentration of 1.8 µg/L: in the upper part of the therapeutic range, but probably necessary since the patient is in acute AF. If the V_d of 7.3 L/kg were used, the calculated dose would be 570 µg, and 500 µg would still be the dose of choice, although the final concentration would be 1.3 µg/L.

(5) Calculate digoxin clearance CL_{dig}:

$$CL_{dig} = 0.06CL_{cr} + 0.05(IBW)$$
$$= 0.06(27) + 0.05(52)$$
$$CL_{dig} = 4.22\,L/h$$

(6) Calculate digoxin maintenance dose (MD) (aim for C_p^{ss} of 1.5 µg/L):

$$MD = \frac{Clearance \times C_p^{ss} \times \tau}{S \times F}$$
$$= \frac{4.22 \times 1.5 \times 24}{1.0 \times 0.63}$$
$$MD = 241\,\mu g/day$$

Thus a dose of 250 µg/day should be recommended.

(7) Calculate half-life:

$$t_{1/2} = 0.693V_d/CL$$
$$= \frac{0.693 \times 284}{4.22}$$
$$t_{1/2} = 46.6\,h$$

$\rightarrow$

> ◗ **CASE STUDY 7.1** (continued)
>
> Time to reach steady-state concentration is about 3.5 times the half-life, i.e. 7 days. Thus the suggestion is to re-assay in 12 days to assess steady-state concentration. If toxicity or lack of effect is suspected, then an earlier sample should be taken.

References/Further reading

Aronson J K, Grahame-Smith D G (1976). Altered distribution of digoxin in renal failure – a cause of digoxin toxicity? *Br J Clin Pharmacol* 3: 1045–1051.

Aronson J K, Grahame-Smith D G, Hallis K F, Hibble A, Wigley F M (1977). Monitoring digoxin therapy; 1. Plasma concentrations and an *in vitro* assay of tissue response. *Br J Clin Pharmacol* 4: 213–221.

Aronson J K, Grahame-Smith D G, Wigley F M (1978). Monitoring digoxin therapy; the use of plasma digoxin concentration measurements in the diagnosis of digoxin toxicity. *Q J Med* 47: 112–113.

Dobbs S M, Mawer G E, Rogers E M, Woodcock B G (1976). Can digoxin dose requirements be predicted? *Br J Clin Pharmacol* 3: 231–237.

Doherty J E, Perkins W H, Flanagan W J (1967). The distribution and concentration of tritiated digoxin in human tissues. *Ann Intern Med* 66: 116–124.

Englund G, Hallberg P, Artursson P, Michaelsson K, Melhus H (2004). Association between the number of co-administered P-glycoprotein inhibitors and serum digoxin levels in patients on therapeutic drug monitoring. *BMC Med* 2: 8.

Ewy G A, Groves B M, Ball M F, *et al.* (1971). Digoxin metabolism in obesity. *Circulation* 44: 810–814.

Goldman S, Probst P, Selzer A, Cohn K (1975). Inefficacy of therapeutic serum levels of digoxin in controlling the ventricular rate in atrial fibrillation. *Am J Cardiol* 35: 651–655.

Greenblatt D J, Duhme D W, Koch-Weser J, Smith T W (1973). Evaluation of digoxin bioavailability in single-dose studies. *N Engl J Med* 289: 651654.

Hartel G, Kyllonen K, Merikallio E, *et al.* (1976). Human serum and myocardial digoxin. *Clin Pharmacol Ther* 19: 153–157.

Hoeschen R J, Cuddy T E (1975). Dose–response relation between therapeutic levels of serum digoxin and systolic time intervals. *Am J Cardiol* 35: 469–472.

Jusko W J, Szefler S J, Goldfarb A L (1974). Pharmacokinetic design of digoxin dosage, regimens in relation to renal function. *J Clin Pharmacol* 14: 525–535.

Koup J R, Greenblatt D J, Jusko W J, Smith T W, Koch-Weser J (1975). Pharmacokinetics of digoxin in normal subjects after intravenous and infusion doses. *J Pharmacokinet Biopharm* 3: 181–192.

Li Wan Po A, Kendall M J (2003). Optimizing digoxin dosage: the long winding road. *J Clin Pharm Ther* 28: 347–348.

Lloyd B L, Greenblatt D J, Allen M D, Harmatz J S, Smith T W (1978). Pharmacokinetics and bioavailability of digoxin capsules, solution and tablets after single and multiple doses. *Am J Cardiol* 42: 129–135.

Maxwell D L, Gilmour-White S K, Hall S R (1989). Digoxin toxicity due to interaction of digoxin with erythromycin. *Br Med J* 298: 572.

Nicholson P W, Dobbs S M, Rodgers E M (1980). Ideal sampling time for drug assays. *Br J Clin Pharmacol* 9: 467–470.

Ohnhaus E, Spring P, Dettli L (1972). Protein binding of digoxin in human serum. *Eur J Clin Pharmacol* 5: 34–36.

Ohnhaus E E, Vozeh S, Nuesch E (1979). Absorption of digoxin in severe right heart failure. *Eur J Clin Pharmacol* 15: 115–120.

Pleasants R A, Williams D M, Porter R S, Gadsden R H Sr (1989). Reassessment of cross-reactivity of spironolactone metabolites with four digoxin immunoassays. *Ther Drug Monit* 11: 200–204.

Redfors A (1972). Plasma digoxin concentration – its relation to digoxin dosage and clinical effects in patients with atrial fibrillation. *Br Heart J* 34: 383–391.

Rengelshausen J, Goggelmann C, Burhenne J, *et al.* (2003). Contribution of increased oral bioavailability and reduced nonglomerular renal clearance of digoxin to the digoxin–clarithromycin interaction. *Br J Clin Pharmacol* 56: 32–38.

Rodin S M, Johnson B F (1988). Pharmacokinetic interactions with digoxin. *Clin Pharmacokinet* 15: 227–244.

Sheiner L B, Rosenberg B, Maranthe V B (1977). Estimation of population characteristics of pharmacokinetic parameters from routine clinical data. *J Pharmacokinet Biopharm* 5: 445–479.

Sheiner L B, Benet L Z, Pagliaro L A (1981). A standard approach to complying clinical pharmacokinetic data. *J Pharmacokinet Biopharm* 9: 59–127.

Smith J W (1973). Digitalis, Part 1. *N Engl J Med* 289: 945–1010.

Stone J, Bentur Y, Zalstein E, Soldin S, Giesbrecht E (1990). Effect of endogenous digoxin-like substances on the interpretation of high concentrations of digoxin in children. *J Paediatr* 117: 321–325.

Vozeh S (1987). Therapeutic drug monitoring of digoxin. *Eur J Clin Pharmacol* 33: 107–108.

Wells T G, Young R A, Kearns G L (1992). Age-related differences in digoxin toxicity and its treatment. *Drug Saf* 7: 135–151.

Williams P J, Lane J, Murray W, Mergener M A, Kamigaki M (1992). Pharmacokinetics of the digoxin–quinidine interaction via mixed-effect modelling. *Clin Pharmacokinet* 22: 66–74.

8

Theophylline

Otto Roman Frey and Wiltrud Probst

Aims and learning outcomes

The aim of this chapter is to encourage students to apply pharmacokinetics and therapeutic drug monitoring to contribute to a safe and effective theophylline therapy.

Learning outcomes for this chapter are:

- To define the actual role of theophylline in asthma and chronic obstructive pulmonary disease.
- To describe the relationship between efficacy, side-effects and drug concentration for theophylline.
- To list the criteria for when it is appropriate to measure theophylline drug concentration.
- To list the factors that modify theophylline pharmacokinetics.
- To calculate the appropriate loading dose and maintenance dose based on population data and measured drug levels.

Rationale for therapeutic drug monitoring (TDM)

The bronchodilatory, anti-inflammatory, immunomodulatory and bronchoprotective effects of theophylline have been applied successfully for many years. Its role in the therapy of asthma and chronic obstructive pulmonary disease (COPD) has been redefined recently. Since the introduction of long-acting inhaled β-agonists, use of theophylline is declining. In patients with moderate to severe asthma who receive inhaled glucocorticoids and β-adrenergic drugs, theophylline should be considered as an additive treatment. When given as a sustained-release preparation, theophylline has a long duration of action and is thus especially useful in the control of nocturnal asthma symptoms. In patients who require maintenance oral corticosteroid therapy, theophylline may be used as a glucocorticoid-sparing agent. The role of intravenously administered theophylline in the treatment of severe acute asthma is controversial. Nevertheless, it should be considered as an additive therapy in all hospitalised patients. In patients with COPD, use of theophylline as a first-line drug therapy may be unreasonable, except in those who are unable to comply with the use of inhaled bronchodilators. If patients' symptoms are not adequately controlled with inhaled β-agonists and anticholinergics, theophylline should be considered. Owing to its broader therapeutic range, caffeine is now preferred over theophylline for the therapy of neonatal apnoea.

Theophylline is associated with severe toxicity, which can usually be observed in concentrations greater than 20 mg/L. Life-threatening effects such as arrhythmias and seizures may occur without any warning signs. Therefore, the great inter- and intraindividual variability of theophylline clearance requires an individual dosage regimen. As it is difficult to adjust theophylline dosage on the basis of clinical response alone, therapeutic drug monitoring is an important element in improving the safety and efficacy of theophylline therapy.

The following characteristics make theophylline suitable for therapeutic drug monitoring:

- Narrow therapeutic index
- Serious toxicities reported
- Known correlation between serum level and toxicity
- Defined therapeutic concentration range
- Significant interpatient variability in pharmacokinetics
- Known factors of clinical relevance that may alter clearance (e.g. concurrent drugs and disease states)

Therapeutic range and evidence-base

Theophylline is an anti-inflammatory drug, even at drug levels of 5–10 mg/L. The bronchodilatory effect of theophylline strongly correlates with the blood level. A linear relationship exists between improvement in pulmonary function and the logarithm of theophylline serum level in the range 5–20 mg/L. Most of the improvement occurs at concentrations of 10 mg/L and less; 65% of the maximum available bronchodilatory effect is achieved with levels of 10 mg/L, whereas higher values reduce response.

The traditionally accepted therapeutic range used to be between 10 and 20 mg/L. Over the last decade, the view of the most appropriate therapeutic range has changed. Today, in order to improve the safety of theophylline therapy by avoiding toxicity, the target range in asthma is stated to be 5–15 mg/L. Serious toxic effects do not occur at concentrations within this range. Any clinical benefit of a theophylline serum level above

15 mg/L has to outweigh the risks. Although no large studies have ever analysed the anti-inflammatory effect of theophylline in COPD, many guidelines recommend a higher level between 10 and 15 mg/L. It has been suggested by other investigators that levels of 8–12 mg/L may be adequate in COPD. Because of reduced protein binding and caffeine being the active metabolite, levels of 5–10 mg/L may be adequate for the treatment of premature apnoea.

> Desired therapeutic range: 5–15 mg/L (28–85 μmol/L)
> Toxic range: >20 mg/L (111 μmol/L)

The majority of side-effects of theophylline are related to serum concentrations and have been reported mostly at levels exceeding 20 mg/L. At levels over 40 mg/L, there is a higher risk of severe events such as seizures and cardiac arrhythmias. Serious toxicity may occur without warning, i.e. not preceded by minor adverse effects. Adverse effects related to theophylline drug levels are listed in Table 8.1.

Table 8.1 Adverse effects related to theophylline drug levels

Theophylline drug serum concentration	Adverse effects	Severity
>10 mg/L	Nausea Insomnia Nervousness Headaches	Minor, mainly transient [a]
>20 mg/L	Nausea Vomiting Diarrhoea Insomnia Irritability Headaches Tremor	Potentially serious
>35 mg/l	Hyperkalaemia Hyperglycaemia Hypotension Hyperthermia Cardiac arrhythmia Cardiorespiratory arrest Cerebral hypoxia with brain injury Seizures Death	Life-threatening

[a] Especially following rapid attainment of a serum level >10 mg/L, the infusion rate should not exceed 20 mg/min.

Theophylline concentrations predict the risk of seizure and cardiac toxicity in both acute and chronic intoxication. As there is often a lag between achieving potentially toxic concentrations and the appearance of a major complication, it has been suggested that these concentrations should be used as an indication to perform extracorporal removal (charcoal haemoperfusion, haemodialysis or haemofiltration) in acute intoxications. Extracorporal removal should be considered at concentrations exceeding 50 mg/L. Patients who have ingested more than 10 mg/kg of theophylline should receive repeated doses of activated charcoal.

Pharmacokinetic profile (ADME)

Absorption

Theophylline is available in a wide range of formulations and different salt forms. The bioavailability (F) of the different products and the salt factor (S) characterise the amount of theophylline administered. Theophylline doses are expressed in terms of anhydrous theophylline. The theophylline salt equivalence of different salts compared to anhydrous theophylline is shown in Table 8.2.

The absorption of theophylline from oral solutions and rapid-release tablets or capsules is rapid and virtually complete. Following ingestion of

Table 8.2 Salt equivalence (S) and bioavailability (F) for different theophylline formulations

Salt form	Anhydrous theophylline content
Aminophylline anhydrous	86%
Aminophylline hydrous	79%
Theophylline monohydrate	91%
Choline theophyllinate	64%
Dosage form	*Bioavailability (F)*
Theophylline IV	100%
Oral liquids	100%
Oral tablets and capsules (immediate release)	100%
Enteric-coated	Delayed, incomplete
Oral tablets and capsules (extended release)	90–100%
Suppositories (cocoa-butter base)	Delayed, incomplete, unpredictable
Rectal solutions	100%

a liquid solution, theophylline can be detected within 10–15 min. Serum concentration curves are similar to those obtained with intravenous administration.

A great number of extended-release products have been formulated in order to prolong the dosing interval of theophylline to 12 and 24 h for chronic therapy. The rate and extent of absorption may differ between various products as well as between different dosages of the same preparation. It is therefore important to refer to the data provided by the manufacturer.

The absorption of theophylline from suppositories is rather slow and unpredictable, which makes dosage regulation difficult and dangerous. The use of theophylline suppositories should be avoided. However, rectal solutions deliver rapid and complete absorption.

Food does not generally reduce the absorption of rapid-release oral theophylline to any important extent. Sustained-release formulations, on the other hand, appear to lead to variable absorption, although the absorption rate and time to peak are more affected than the extent of drug absorption. Reduced theophylline blood levels were noted in patients receiving enteral tube feeding.

Distribution

Theophylline distributes rapidly in the extracellular fluid. Further distribution sites are breast milk, cerebrospinal fluid, saliva (65% of serum), and other body secretions.

The total protein binding is about 40% in adults and children. This rate may be as low as 30–35% in patients with hepatic cirrhosis, in those with reduced serum albumin concentration, and in neonates. As the general protein binding of theophylline is low, these changes are not clinically significant. However, in a few selected situations, measurement of free theophylline levels may be helpful.

The apparent volume of distribution (V_d) averages about 0.5 L/kg in healthy children and adults and ranges from 0.3 to 0.7 L/kg. It is slightly higher in premature infants, in adults with hepatic cirrhosis, and in patients suffering from uncorrected acidaemia. It may be lower in adults with COPD, in elderly patients, and in patients with uncorrected alkaemia. The interindividual variability of the volume of distribution in relation to body weight is low in comparison with theophylline clearance, which is affected by many factors. The volume of distribution itself is not affected by an altered clearance. In calculating the volume of distribution, ideal body weight (IBW) should be used.

Metabolism

Theophylline is predominantly (85–90%) metabolised via hepatic bio-transformation. Theophylline is N-demethylated to 3-methylxanthine and 1-methylxanthine by the cytochrome system P450 1A2 (53%). Hydroxylation in the C-8 position (40%) by cytochrome P450 2E1 and 3A3 leads to 1,3-dimethyluric acid as the major metabolite. These metabolites are relatively inactive. The only active one, 3-methyltheophylline, is rather irrelevant. As the activity of the 1A2 isoenzyme is reduced in the elderly and still undeveloped in neonates, the hepatic metabolism is age-related, with rapid changes occurring in the first year of life and a decrease in the elderly (see p. 155). Owing to the differences in the rate of metabolism, half-lives of theophylline show a wide interpatient variation, ranging from 3 to 30 h. The mean half-life in nonsmoking (healthy) adults is assumed to be 8 h.

In some patients, the metabolism of theophylline is saturable, and dosage adjustment can result in disproportionately large changes in serum concentration.

Elimination

Differences in the rate of hepatic metabolism result in a great variability of theophylline clearance. Numerous factors can decrease theophylline elimination, e.g. age, disease and concurrent drugs with a potential to interact. Smoking increases theophylline elimination, which is why smokers require a high daily dosage. These factors are described in more detail on p. 157. Less than 10% of theophylline is excreted unchanged via the urine, so that renal dysfunction does not require dosage adjustment.

Population data

Table 8.3 summarises the mean pharmacokinetic parameters of theophylline in various populations. The values are based on different sources and personal experiences, and can be used to estimate individual parameters.

Equation resource

$$IBW_{male} = 50 + [height \ (cm) - 152.4] \times 0.89 \ (kg) \qquad (8.1)$$

$$D = \Delta C_p \times V_d \qquad (8.2)$$

$$k = \frac{\ln(C_2/C_1)}{\Delta t} \tag{8.3}$$

$$t_{1/2} = \frac{\ln 2}{k} \tag{8.4}$$

$$t_{1/2} = \frac{\ln 2 \times V_d}{CL} \tag{8.5}$$

$$C_p^{ss} = \frac{F \times S \times D}{\tau \times CL} \tag{8.6}$$

$$t_{max} = \frac{\ln(k_a/k)}{k_a - k} \tag{8.7}$$

$$C_{pt} = \frac{F \times S \times D \times k_a}{V_d(k_a - k)} \times \left[\frac{\exp(-kt)}{1 - \exp(-k\tau)} - \frac{\exp(-k_a t)}{1 - \exp(-k_a \tau)} \right] \tag{8.8}$$

$$C_{pt} = C_p \exp(-kt) \tag{8.9}$$

Table 8.3 Mean pharmacokinetic parameters of theophylline in various populations

	Mean clearance		Mean volume of distribution (L)	Mean half-life (h)
	(L/h/kg)	(mL/min/kg)		
Premature neonates	0.017	0.28	0.8	30
Term neonates	0.019	0.32	0.7	25
Infants 1–5 months	0.048	0.8	0.7	11
Infants 6–12 months	0.120	2.0	0.7	4,6
Children 1–3 years	0.102	1.7	0.6	3,4
Children 4–15 years	0.090	1.5	0.5	3,8
Adults 16–60 years	0.039	0.65	0.5	8
Elderly >60 years	0.025	0.42	0.4	11

Reason for request

Plasma level monitoring of theophylline is a particularly useful adjunct to clinical monitoring and is advised:

- When toxicity is suspected (e.g. nausea, vomiting, diarrhoea, pulse >100 bpm, nervousness, agitation, seizures, arrhythmia)
- When a toxic serum level declines

- When efficacy is questioned
- When compliance is questioned
- Before giving a loading dose in case of a pre-existing theophylline drug level
- Sometimes approximately 1 h after administration of the loading dose to verify the concentration and to allow calculation of the infusion dose
- To ensure steady-state concentration after 5 half-lives
- When other drugs that are known to alter theophylline clearance, are added or subtracted
- When conditions have developed that are known to alter theophylline clearance (e.g. febrile illness, pregnancy, liver disease, congestive heart failure, smoking cessation)
- When enteral tube feeding is begun or stopped
- When route of administration or formulation of theophylline are changed.

Following the establishment of the dosage regimen that maintains serum concentrations within the therapeutic range, dosage requirements normally remain stable for extended periods. For this reason, the need for measuring blood levels routinely at regular intervals in adults is controversial. In children, however, growth effectively results in a decrease of the weight-adjusted dose and repeated measurements may be needed as frequently as every 6 months. Monitoring should be done on trough specimens after steady state has been reached. Non-steady-state concentrations may be indicated in the particular situations mentioned above.

Factors affecting drug levels, including important drug interactions

Theophylline is eliminated via various pathways. Approximately 10% is eliminated unchanged through the kidneys. Ninety per cent of ingested theophylline is transformed by the hepatic microsomal enzymes (CYP1A2, CYP2E1, CYP3A3) into at least four major metabolites, which are also excreted by the kidney. While renal function does not affect theophylline levels, altered hepatic function has a significant influence on theophylline clearance. Theophylline interacts with numerous drugs (Table 8.4), but not all well-known inhibitors of drug metabolism affect theophylline. When starting *and* when discontinuing interacting drugs, theophylline serum concentrations should be monitored to adjust dosage, and the time course of interaction should be observed. If possible, interactions

Table 8.4 Selected drug–drug interactions

Drug	Mean effect on theophylline clearance (CL)
Allopurinol	CL ↓ ~25%
Aminoglutethimide	CL ↓ ~25%
Barbiturates	CL ↑ ~25%
Carbamazepine	CL ↑ ~50 %
Cimetidine	CL ↓ ~40%
Ciprofloxacin	CL ↓ ~40%
Clarithromycin	CL ↓ ~25%
Diltiazem	CL ↓ ~20%
Disulfiram	CL ↓ ~25%
Enoxacin	CL ↓ ~40%
Erythromycin	CL ↓ ~25%
Felodipine	CL ↑ ~20%
Fluvoxamine	CL ↓ ~50%
Interferon	CL ↓ ~50%
Isoniazid	CL ↓ ~25%
Isoprenaline	CL ↓ ~20%
Methotrexate	CL ↓ ~20%
Norfloxacin	CL ↓ ~15%
Ofloxacin	CL ↓ ~10%
Oral contraceptives	CL ↓ ~30%
Phenylpropanolamine	CL ↓ ~50%
Phenytoin	CL ↑ ~75%
Propafenone	CL ↓ ~40%
Propranolol	CL ↓ ~30%
Rifampicin	CL ↑ ~50%
Ticlopidine	CL ↓ ~40%
Terbutaline	CL ↑ ~20%
Verapamil	CL ↓ ~20%
Viloxazine	CL ↓ ~50%

should be circumvented by choosing an alternative drug, e.g. ranitidine instead of cimetidine or azithromycin instead of erythromycin.

Moreover, there are several diseases that may alter serum theophylline concentrations. Other factors to be considered are the patient's age, ideal body weight, diet and smoking history. Although young children metabolise theophylline faster than adults, clearance is markedly decreased in newborns. Cigarette smoking usually improves theophylline clearance; within 1 week after cessation of smoking, theophylline elimination may be slowed by more than 30%, and full recovery may take several months (Table 8.5). High-protein diets may increase elimination, and high-carbohydrate diets may reduce the loss of theophylline from the body.

Table 8.5 Selected drug–disease or drug–condition interactions

Disease/condition	Mean effect on theophylline clearance (CL)
Acute pulmonary oedema	CL ↓ ~50%
Congestive heart failure	CL ↓ ~40%
Cor pulmonale	CL ↓ ~40%
Cystic fibrosis	CL ↑ ~100%
Hyperthyroidism	CL ↑ ~25%
Liver cirrhosis	CL ↓ ~40%
Pneumonia (febrile)	CL ↓ ~25%
Viral hepatitis	CL ↓ ~40%
Passive smoking	CL ↑ ~25%
Mild smoking	CL ↑ ~50%
Heavy smoking	CL ↑ ~100%
Cannabis smoking	CL ↑ ~50%

Theophylline is distributed throughout the body water. The mean volume of distribution in premature infants, in adults with hepatic cirrhosis or in uncorrected acidaemia is slightly larger. In all other circumstances V_d remains unaffected, and a value of 0.5 L/kg can be assumed. In obese patients, ideal body weight should be used for calculation. The bioavailability of theophylline can be increased or decreased by food in general and by the type of food eaten in particular. Marked changes in bioavailability of theophylline can occur in patients receiving nasogastric tube feeding.

A careful evaluation of the patient's history is recommended before starting theophylline therapy. Changes in lifestyle, disease and medication must be monitored during therapy in order to prevent intoxication or loss of efficacy.

Clinical case studies

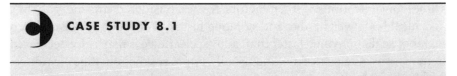

CASE STUDY 8.1

M.H. is a 56-year-old man (98 kg, 177 cm). He is admitted to hospital on Saturday evening at 1900 h suffering from acute respiratory distress. M.H. has

→

a 30-year history of asthma. As his wife reports, the asthma has been reasonably well controlled by the following medications over the last 2 years:

Beclometasone	*inhaled 2 times daily*
Salmeterol	*inhaled 2 times daily*
Theophylline (extended release)	*350 mg every 12 hours*

His wife further reports that her husband missed the last three doses of each medication because he had been suffering from a severe headache over the last two days.

As M.H. does not respond well to inhaled β-agonists and systemic cortico-steroids, and because a theophylline concentration of 3.0 mg/L is measured, an additional loading dose is ordered.

Recommend an appropriate loading dose of theophylline to reach a serum level of 12 mg/L

The theophylline loading dose is determined from its apparent volume of distribution, which is 0.5 L/kg on average in adults. In obese patients, ideal body weight (IBW) should be used to calculate V_d (equation 8.1):

$$IBW_{male} = [50 + [height (cm) - 152.4] \times 0.89] (kg)$$

With an IBW of 72 kg, the absolute volume of distribution for M.H. is 72 × 0.5 L/kg = 36 L. To elevate the theophylline serum level from 3 to 12 mg/L, the loading dose can be calculated with equation (8.2):

$$D = \Delta C_p \times V_d$$

9 mg/L × 36 L = 324 mg theophylline (410 mg aminophylline)

A loading dose of 400 mg aminophylline is recommended.

M.H. receives the calculated loading dose as a 30-min infusion. Therapy is continued by continuous infusion of 600 mg aminophylline diluted in 500 mL glucose 5% (infusion rate 30 mg/h). His symptoms improve over the following 1–2 h. During the night he complains of restlessness, insomnia and nausea. At 0300 h, a theophylline drug level of 28 mg/L (5–15; toxic > 20 mg/L) is measured and reported to the ward. The theophylline infusion is stopped immediately.

Are M.H.'s symptoms consistent with theophylline toxicity? What other adverse effects might be caused by theophylline overdosing?

Restlessness, insomnia and nausea are common adverse effects of theophylline associated with drug levels exceeding 20 mg/L. Further effects that have been reported include vomiting, diarrhoea, irritability, headache, tachycardia, arrhythmia and seizures.

→

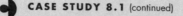

CASE STUDY 8.1 (continued)

What might be the reason for the high theophylline level?
Within 7 h, an additional 210 mg of aminophylline (166 mg theophylline) was
administered to M.H. Even if no theophylline was metabolised, an increase
from 3 mg/L to 28 mg/L by application of 610 mg aminophylline (482 mg
theophylline) seems to be impossible. Other reasons for the observed intoxication may be an error in measuring or reporting the level in the evening or a
medication error on the ward.

In this case, M.H. admits that when he started to become short of breath in
the afternoon, he took a few doses of theophylline that he had skipped earlier.
As the absorption of the extended-release formulations is prolonged, the symptoms did not improve. While theophylline was administered by infusion, the
extended-release theophylline was slowly absorbed at the same time and led
to the toxic drug level. A careful drug history should always be taken in order
to know how much theophylline has been administered over the previous 48 h.

At 1100 h, the theophylline level is measured again and reported to be
12.8 mg/L. The symptoms have improved, and the route of administration should
be changed to oral.

**Suggest an appropriate maintenance dosing regimen for M.H. Calculate
clearance on the basis of the two theophylline levels measured and the
average volume of distribution (population data). The bioavailability of the
extended-release tablets is assumed to be 90%, the achieved mean steady-
state concentration should be 8 mg/L.**
Assuming that no more theophylline is absorbed after 0300 h, k_e and the individual half-life can be calculated using equations (8.3) and (8.4):

$$k = \frac{\ln(C_2/C_1)}{\Delta t}$$
$$k = 0.0978 \text{ h}^{-1}$$

$$t_{1/2} = \frac{\ln 2}{k}$$
$$t_{1/2} = 7.1 \text{ h}$$

To calculate maintenance dose, equations (8.5) and (8.6) can be used:

$$t_{1/2} = \frac{\ln 2 \times V_d}{CL}$$

→

> **CASE STUDY 8.1** (continued)

Assuming a V_d of 36 L and a half-life of 7.1 h, theophylline clearance of M.H. equals 3.5 L/h.

$$C_p^{ss} = \frac{F \times S \times D}{\tau \times CL}$$

To achieve a C_p^{ss} of 8 mg/L, a dose of 31 mg/h or 744 mg/day theophylline divided in two doses is recommended. In practice, M.H. may receive his previous dose of 350 mg two times daily.

$$D \times S \times F/\tau = CL \times C_{p\,ave}^{ss}$$
$$F = 0.9$$
$$D \times S = \frac{3.5 \times 8}{0.9} = 31 \text{ mg/h of theophylline}$$
$$D \times S = 744 \text{ mg/day theophylline}$$
$$= 942 \text{ mg/day aminophylline}$$
$$= 450 \text{ mg two times daily of Phyllocontin}$$
$$\text{(aminophylline SR)}$$

> **CASE STUDY 8.2**

A.T. is a 46-year-old male (63 kg/176 cm) with a long history of COPD, currently treated with tiotropium 18 µg daily, salmeterol 50 µg 2 times daily and salbutamol 100 µg as required. He is still smoking 5–10 cigarettes per day. Because of decreased exercise tolerance and increasing shortness of breath, theophylline is added to his therapy.

What is the therapeutic range of theophylline in COPD?
In general, the therapeutic range of theophylline is 5–15 mg/L. However, some guidelines recommend levels of 10–15 mg/L, whereas some other investigators have suggested that it might be adequate to attain levels of 8–12 mg/L in COPD.

$\rightarrow$

> **CASE STUDY 8.2** (continued)

What dosing regimen do you recommend to achieve a mean steady-state concentration of 10 mg/L? (Theophylline extended-release capsules: 100, 350 or 500 mg theophylline monohydrate; $k_a = 0.2\,h^{-1}$; $F = 0.85$)

The theophylline clearance of A.T. is increased by smoking at a factor of approximately 1.5%. Thus a clearance of 0.039 L/h/kg (population data) × 1.5 (mild smoking factor) = 0.0585 L/h/kg and a total clearance of 0.0585 × 63 kg = 3.7 L/h can be assumed.

Equation (8.6) is used to calculate the daily dose ($F = 0.85$ (bioavailability), $S = 0.91$ (salt factor), $\tau = 24$ h, CL = 3.7 L/h):

$$C_p^{ss} = \frac{F \times S \times D}{\tau \times CL}$$

$$D = 48\ mg/h\ or\ 1152\ mg/24\ h$$

A dose of 1000 mg/24 h seems to be suitable; slow-release formulations are usually administered in two separate doses. A starting dose of 500 mg every 12 h can be recommended.

What time to maximum concentration, t_{max}, and which concentrations 1 h, 8 h and 12 h following intake are expected in steady state?

Equation (8.5) is used to calculate $t_{1/2}$ and k ($V_d = 63$ kg × 0.5 L/kg = 31.5 L; CL = 3.7 L/h):

$$t_{1/2} = \frac{\ln 2 \times V_d}{CL}$$

$$t_{1/2} = 5.9\ h$$
$$k = 0.1175\ h^{-1}$$

and equation (8.7) is used to calculate t_{max} ($k_a = 0.20\,h^{-1}$):

$$t_{max} = \frac{\ln(k_a/k)}{k_a - k}$$

Maximum concentration is expected to be reached 6.4 h following ingestion of theophylline extended-release capsules.

To calculate concentrations following administration of oral formulations, equation (8.8) is used ($F = 0.85$; $S = 0.91$; $D = 500$ mg; $k_a = 0.20\,h^{-1}$; $k = 0.1175\,h^{-1}$; $V_d = 31.5$ L; $\tau = 12$ h; CL = 3.7 L/h):

$$C_{pt} = \frac{F \times S \times D \times k_a}{V_d(k_a - k)} \times \left[\frac{\exp(-kt)}{1 - \exp(-k\tau)} - \frac{\exp(-k_a t)}{1 - \exp(-k_a \tau)} \right]$$

$\rightarrow$

⬤ **CASE STUDY 8.2** (continued)

C_{1h} = 8.2 mg/L

C_{8h} = 8.8 mg/L

C_{12h} = 6.6 mg/L

When should the first blood sample be taken?
A short half-life of 5.9 h is expected in A.T. Steady-state conditions are reached within 24–30 h after starting therapy. A trough level measurement before the fourth dose can be recommended.

The measured theophylline level is 8 mg/L. What recommendations would you make?
The theophylline concentration lies within the therapeutic range. If adequate effects are achieved, no change in dosing is required.

Because of problems swallowing the tablets, A.T. is converted to theophylline solution (theophylline monohydrate; k_a = 3.5 h^{-1}; F = 1.0, S = 0.91). What influence on t_{max}, and concentrations 1 h and 12 h following intake are expected, and what are your recommendations?
Equation (8.7) is used to calculate t_{max}; to calculate concentrations following administration of oral formulations, equation (8.8) is used (F = 1.0; S = 0.91; D = 500 mg; k_a = 3.5 h^{-1}, k = 0.1175 h^{-1}; $t_{1/2}$ = 5.9 h; V_d = 31.5 L; τ = 12 h; CL = 3.7 L/h):

$$t_{max} = \frac{\ln(k_a/k)}{k_a - k}$$

$$C_{pt} = \frac{F \times S \times D \times k_a}{V_d(k_a - k)} \times \left[\frac{\exp(-kt)}{1 - \exp(-k\tau)} - \frac{\exp(-k_a t)}{1 - \exp(-k_a \tau)} \right]$$

t_{max} = 1 h

C_{1h} = 17.1 mg/L

C_{12h} = 4.4 mg/L

Oral solutions of theophylline are absorbed rapidly. Changing from slow-release formulations to solutions carries the risk of a wide fluctuation of serum levels between doses. After ingestion, side-effects such as tachycardia or vomiting can occur. Dosing interval must be reduced to 4–6 h. For A.T. capsules with slow-release pellets would be a suitable alternative.

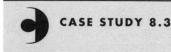

CASE STUDY 8.3

R.T., a 42-year-old man (184 cm, 68 kg) with COPD, is admitted to hospital because of an acute exacerbation. At day 4, a blood sample is drawn because of suspected theophylline toxicity. The concentration 12 h following intake is 30 mg/L and 4 h later is 25 mg/L.

	Previous medication	Since admission
Metoprolol	190 mg/day	
Aspirin	100 mg/day	
Ipratropium/fenoterol	4 puffs/day	8 puffs/day
Theophylline (S = 1.0; F = 0.9; k_a = 0.3 h^{-1})	500 mg every 12 h	500 mg every 8 h
Ranitidine		300 mg/day
Erythromycin		1000 mg every 8 h

What reasons for the intoxication can you find?
No drug level was drawn on admission. Even if the theophylline level of A.T. was within the lower therapeutic range, increasing dosage by 50% is not recommended. Additionally, application of erythromycin can markedly decrease theophylline clearance. In contrast to cimetidine, ranitidine does not affect the pharmacokinetics of theophylline.

What current theophylline half-life can be calculated?
Using equations (8.3) and (8.4):

$$k = \frac{\ln(C_2/C_1)}{\Delta t}$$
$$k = 0.0456 \text{ h}^{-1}$$

$$t_{1/2} = \frac{\ln 2}{k}$$
$$t_{1/2} = 15.2 \text{ h}$$

What serum theophylline level do you expect 20 h later?
Using equation (8.9) (C_0 = 25 mg/L; k = 0.0456 h^{-1}; t = 20 h):

$$C_{pt} = C_p \exp(-kt)$$

a serum theophylline level of about 10 mg/L is expected.

$\rightarrow$

CASE STUDY 8.3 (continued)

What dosing regimen do you recommend to achieve a C_p^{ss} of 10 mg/L?

Assuming $t_{1/2}$ = 15.2 h and V_d = 0.5 L/kg × 68 kg = 34 L, using equation (8.5)

$$t_{1/2} = \frac{\ln 2 \times V_d}{CL}$$

a clearance of 1.55 L/h can be calculated.

To calculate the daily dose, equation (8.6) is used (F = 0.9 (bioavailability), S = 1 (salt factor), τ = 24 h, CL = 1.55 L/h):

$$C_p^{ss} = \frac{F \times S \times D}{\tau \times CL}$$
$$D = 17 \text{ mg/h or } 408 \text{ mg/24 h}$$

A dose of 400 mg/24 h seems to be suitable. Slow-release formulations are usually administered in two separate doses; 200 mg every 12 h can be recommended.

What are your recommendations concerning theophylline dosage and blood sampling?

Measurement of the drug level is recommended after 20–24 h. If the level has decreased to the expected range, 200 mg every 12 h should be started. It is advisable to check the serum level 48 h later. Theophylline clearance will improve following discontinuation of antibiotic therapy, and theophylline levels may fall below the therapeutic range.

CASE STUDY 8.4

A.K., an 82-year-old woman (48 kg), is admitted to hospital. She is diagnosed as having an ischaemic stroke. Over the next three days, her neurological status improves, and her previous medications should be given again. As A.K. is still not able to swallow well, nasogastric tube feeding is continued, and medication should be administered via the tube. A.K. has a long history of chronic obstructive pulmonary disease; laboratory analyses revealed a serum creatinine of 140 μmol/L.

→

🌓 **CASE STUDY 8.4** (continued)

> *Her previous medications were:*
> *Theophylline (extended release; $S = 1$; $F = 0.9$; $k_a = 0.25 h^{-1}$)*
>   *200 mg o.d.*
> *Fluticasone*   *2 puffs per day*
> *Salbutamol*   *2 puffs per day*
> *Allopurinol*   *300 mg o.d.*
> *Enalapril*   *10 mg b.d.*
> *Bendroflumethiazide*   *2.5 mg o.d.*

The pharmacist was asked to propose a suitable theophylline formulation compatible with tube feeding. What would you recommend?
In general, extended-release formulations should not be crushed. They could be changed to rapid-release formulations, liquids or tablets that can be crushed, or capsules that can be opened and administered via the tube. The dosing interval has to be adjusted regarding the formulation and the patient's clearance. For A.K., the daily dose can be divided into two doses. Alternatively, rectal solutions might be suitable, apart from suppositories because of the unpredictable absorption of theophylline.

Why is theophylline drug monitoring indicated?
If dosage or formulation is changed, drug level monitoring is recommended. Additionally, concurrent enteral tube feeding can decrease theophylline serum level. Starting and discontinuing enteral feeding are indications for theophylline monitoring.

Are there any specific theophylline dosage recommendation for elderly people? Does theophylline needs any adjustment in patients with renal failure? Is there any other factor that can affect A.K.'s clearance?
In the elderly, age-related alteration in theophylline hepatic metabolism may occur. Therefore, the relatively low theophylline dosage may be suitable for A.K. Dosage is adjusted with the aid of drug monitoring and clinical efficacy. In general, the theophylline dose needs no adjustment in renal failure. Additionally, the co-medication of allopurinol can decrease theophylline clearance by about 25%. When a prolonged half-life is assumed (elderly, allopurinol), a liquid formulation and a dosage of 100 mg two times daily can be recommended.

What is the expected mean theophylline concentration in steady state? When should the blood sample be taken at the earliest, and what sampling time do you propose?
The theophylline level measured is 3.8 mg/L.

→

> ● **CASE STUDY 8.4** (continued)
>
> To calculate the expected mean steady-state concentration, equation (8.6) is used ($F = 0.9$ (bioavailability); $S = 1$ (salt factor); $CL = 0.025 \times 0.75$ (factor allopurinol) $\times 48\,kg = 0.9\,L/h$, $D = 200\,mg$, $\tau = 24\,h$):
>
> $$C_p^{ss} = \frac{F \times S \times D}{\tau \times CL}$$
>
> Expected $C_p^{ss} = 8.3\,mg/L$.
> The theophylline drug level should be monitored when steady state has been achieved.
> Assuming $CL = 0.9\,L/h$ and $V_d = 0.4\,L/kg \times 48\,kg = 19.2\,L$ and using equation (8.5):
>
> $$t_{1/2} = \frac{\ln 2 \times V_d}{CL}$$
>
> a half-life of 14.8 h can be calculated. Steady state will be reached within 3 days (4–5 times the half-life). The pre-dose (trough) level should be measured, for example in the morning.
>
> **What recommendations would you make concerning the following theophylline dosage?**
> The measured trough level lies below the expected level and the therapeutic range. Tube feeding may have decreased the theophylline level.
> Dosage should be adjusted. As a first step, an increase to 125 mg every 12 hours is recommended.

References/Further reading

Darsey E H (2001). Theophylline. In: Murphy J E, ed. *Clinical Pharmacokinetics*, 2nd edn. Bethesda MD: ASHP Publications Production Centre, 345–360.

Global Initiative for Asthma website (1995 revised 2004). *Global Initiative for Asthma. Global Strategy for Asthma Management and Prevention*. Bethesda MD: NHLB/WHO (www.guideline.gov).

Hendeles L, Weinberger M (1983). Theophylline – A "state of the art" review. *Pharmacotherapy* 3(1): 2–42.

McEvoy G K, ed. (2001). Theophyllines. *American Hospital Formulary Service Drug Information*. Bethesda MD: American Society of Health-System Pharmacists, 3483–3490.

Ohnishi A, Kato M, Kojima J, Ushiama H, Yoneko M, Kawai H (2003). Differential pharmacokinetics of theophylline in elderly patients. *Drugs Aging* 20(1): 71–84.

Self T H, Heilker G M, Alloway R R, Kelso T M, Abou-Shala N (1993). Reassessing the therapeutic range for theophylline on laboratory report forms: the importance of 5–15 µg/ml. *Pharmacotherapy* 13(6): 590–594.

Upton R A (1991). Pharmacokinetic interactions between theophylline and other medication (part I) and (part II). *Clin Pharmacokinet* 20: 66–80, 135–150.

Vassallo R, Lipsky J S (1998). Theophylline: recent advances in the understanding of its mode of action and uses in clinical practice. *Mayo Clin Proc* 73: 346–354.

9

Lithium

Patricia M Morgan

Aims and learning outcomes

The aims of this chapter are:

- To place the therapeutic drug monitoring of lithium in the clinical setting.
- To provide the information necessary for its safe use.
- To highlight the potential dangers of lithium in the course of treatment.

Introduction

Lithium is unique as a therapeutic entity. The lightest of all the solid elements in the Periodic Table with an atomic weight of 3, it is widely prevalent in food and water and has become one of the most researched and written about drugs in medical history, yet its mode of action in manic depression (bipolar disorder) is still not fully understood.

Lithium is licensed for the treatment of mania, prevention of relapse in manic depression illness, treatment of recurrent depression and management of aggressive or self-mutilating behaviour. Lithium and clozapine are the only drugs shown to decrease the risk of suicide in bipolar disorder and schizophrenia, respectively. Because of the potential risks (narrow therapeutic range and discontinuation), lithium should only be started by a specialist and needs to be continued for at least two years to be beneficial. The likely duration of treatment should be discussed with the patient before treatment begins and treatment should not be started unless the patient seems likely to adhere to therapy and blood testing. Shorter durations, rapid discontinuation and erratic compliance increase the risk of adverse outcomes.

Mode of action

Since the discovery of its therapeutic effects, lithium has been shown to act on multiple sites. Recent molecular studies have revealed the action of lithium on signal transduction mechanisms such as phosphinositide (PI) hydrolysis, adenylyl cyclase, G protein, glycogen synthase kinase 3β (GSK-3β) and protein kinase C (PKC) and its substrate myristoylated alanine-rich C kinase substrate (MARCKS).

There are multiple abnormalities in neurotransmitters in bipolar disorder and it is unclear whether these are independent or there is an overriding dysfunctional control mechanism. Postulated modes of action of lithium can be divided into four categories (though this is a gross over-simplification), with effects on:

- First-messengers systems: dopamine, serotonin, noradrenaline, acetylcholine, γ-aminobutyric acid (GABA), glutamate
- Second messengers and neuropeptides: G proteins, adenylyl cyclase pump, PI
- Ion transfer, replacing sodium, potassium, calcium and magnesium
- Gene expression and neuroplasticity: Bcl-2 upregulation, GSK-3β inhibition, resulting in neuroprotective and neurotrophic effects

Thus, 'analogous to a conductor, lithium orchestrates an altered pattern of signalling throughout critical regions on the brain' (Lenox and Hahn, 2000). Its mode of action may be any of the above, or a combination, or none.

The most extraordinary discovery about lithium in recent times is its neurotrophic effects. Lithium has been demonstrated to inhibit GSK-3β, an enzyme known to regulate the levels of phosphorylated tau protein and β-catenin (both of which may play a role in the neurodegeneration observed in Alzheimer disease). These findings suggest that lithium may exert some of its long-term beneficial effects in the treatment of mood disorders via under-appreciated neuroprotective effects. To date, lithium remains the only medication demonstrated to markedly increase neuro-protective Bcl-2 levels in several brain areas. Investigation of the therapeutic potential of lithium in treating certain long-term neurodegenerative disorders may be warranted.

Rationale for therapeutic drug monitoring (TDM)

Lithium has the narrowest therapeutic index of any medication routinely prescribed in psychiatry and is poorly tolerated in a third or more of treated patients, resulting in a high incidence of noncompliance. The safe/optimal use of lithium requires the application of TDM to control for lithium toxicity. TDM serves also as a test for adherence to the prescribed regimen in the light of other factors that may affect serum concentration, but it is not an ideal method of minimising lithium-induced side-effects.

Initial adverse effects of lithium therapy include nausea, diarrhoea, vertigo, muscle weakness, and a dazed feeling; these effects often abate with continued therapy. Fine hand tremors, polyuria and polydipsia may persist, however. Other adverse effects that may occur at therapeutic serum-lithium concentrations include weight gain, oedema and leucocytosis. Hypercalcaemia, hypermagnesaemia and hyperparathyroidism have been reported. Skin disorders such as acne, psoriasis and rashes may be exacerbated by lithium therapy.

Long-term adverse effects include hypothyroidism and/or goitre, rarely hyperthyroidism, and mild cognitive and memory impairment, although the last has not been distinguished as purely lithium-related in the absence of mood disorder. Histological and functional changes in the kidney are rare and the risk of renal damage and impaired glomerular filtration rate is thought to be extremely small in patients on stable maintenance lithium therapy without prior episodes of acute lithium intoxication. Neurotoxicity is a potential long-term adverse effect that, if minor, can be minimised by a reduction of lithium dose, but if severe warrants discontinuation and complete withdrawal of the drug. Serious effects might include deteriorating cognition and mental status, gait disturbances, movement disorders such as choreoathetosis and myoclonus, seizures and cerebellar signs.

Toxic effects may be expected at serum-lithium concentrations over 1.5 mmol/L, although they can appear at lower concentrations. Signs of lithium toxicity include increasing diarrhoea, vomiting, anorexia, muscle weakness, lethargy, giddiness with ataxia, lack of coordination, tinnitus, blurred vision, coarse tremor of the extremities and lower jaw, muscle hyperirritability, choreoathetoid movements, dysarthria and drowsiness.

Organ toxicity is often encountered when serum concentrations exceed 1.5 mmol/L and life-threatening intoxication with serum concentrations over 3.5 mmol/L.

Symptoms of serious overdosage at serum-lithium concentrations above 2 mmol/L include hyperreflexia and hyperextension of limbs, syncope, toxic psychosis, seizures, polyuria, renal failure, electrolyte imbalance, dehydration, circulatory failure, coma, and occasionally death.

Therapeutic range

Serum lithium concentrations between 0.4 and 1.2 mmol/L (with 0.6–1.0 mmol/L the optimal for maintenance) are generally adhered to as the window within which the highest probability of therapeutic response without serious complications is obtained. In this therapeutic window there are exceptions to the serum concentration–effect relationship and it is important to realise that attainment of serum lithium concentrations within this range does not ensure response in about 20–30% of patients for who lithium is indicated. Some people experience adverse effects from lower levels. Capillary blood samples can be used in 'near-patient' testing using the ion-specific electrode as only 0.1 mL of whole blood is required for the test.

Erythrocyte measurements of lithium have been postulated as a better indicator of intracellular lithium, and the erythrocyte:plasma lithium concentration ratio is a possible indicator of response and toxicity. These results have been inconclusive, however, and so erythrocyte lithium concentrations have relatively limited use in clinical practice (Winter, 1996).

Salivary lithium has also been examined with a view to monitoring without the need for venepuncture. There is a considerable interpatient variability in the serum:saliva ratio, although once this is established for the individual a salivary lithium measurement could be used for patients who have difficulty in giving a venous blood sample. Other methods of testing are atomic emission flame photometry and atomic absorption flame spectrophotometry; both more demanding and slower than the ion-specific electrode.

Relationship of serum concentration measurements to response

There are individual differences in pharmacodynamics and pharmacokinetics as regards distribution of lithium to its sites of action in the CNS. The assumption that circulating lithium reflects the concentration of lithium at extracellular sites of action in the CNS is the basis for therapeutic drug monitoring, but *in vivo* lithium brain imaging techniques have shown brain/serum concentration ratios of between 0.1 and 1.0 during prolonged lithium administration. This explains the substantial interindividual differences in brain lithium at similar serum lithium concentrations.

The practice of therapeutic drug monitoring has enabled widespread clinical use of lithium. This is in part due to the unique pharmacokinetic properties of lithium. Lithium exhibits negligible binding to plasma proteins, does not undergo biotransformation, and is eliminated virtually exclusively by the renal route. These properties greatly simplify the impact of individual pharmacokinetic differences.

Therapeutic drug monitoring, although an essential part of lithium therapy, should therefore be interpreted only in the light of clinical response and emergent adverse effects. One must 'Treat the patient, not the level'.

Therapeutic range and evidence-base

Despite the unique pharmacokinetic profile of lithium in reaching its target site of action in the brain, serum (or plasma) concentration measurement remains the accepted method for optimising dosage. The accepted therapeutic ranges, depending on the indication, are shown in Table 9.1.

Acute mania

Lithium remains a first-line treatment in the treatment of acute mania until formal studies show otherwise (Fraser *et al.*, 2001; Goodwin, 2003) but has the problem that final outcomes are likely to be worse with treatment for less than 2 years. However, some patients do not tolerate typical anti-manic lithium levels. Plasma lithium concentrations up to 1.5 mmol/L may be required in the short term, with doses reduced to achieve 0.8–1.2 mmol/L once mood is stabilised. Time to remission of symptoms appears to be strongly related to rapid achievement of therapeutic drug

Table 9.1 Therapeutic ranges for lithium depending on the indication

Indication	Therapeutic range for samples taken 12–16 h following the preceding dose
Controlling acute mania	Initially up to 1.5 mmol/L may required in the short term, reducing to 0.8–1.2 mmol/L as mood is stabilised
Prophylaxis of bipolar disorder	0.4–1.0 mmol/L (It is important to determine the optimum range for each individual, as patients can respond above, below or within a small band of the range.)
Augmentation of antidepressants in treatment-resistant depression	≥0.5 mmol/L
Aggressive or self-mutilating behaviour	0.4–1.0 mmol/L

levels. The onset of action is 5–7 days or longer, and adjunctive treatment with benzodiazepines and antipsychotic drugs is usually necessary.

Prophylaxis of bipolar disorder

The effectiveness of lithium as a long-term maintenance treatment of mood disorders has been the subject of systematic reviews (Burgess *et al.*, 2003). Baldessarini and Tondo (2000) reviewed the medical literature from 1970 to 1996 and found no indication that benefits from lithium treatment in bipolar disorder have decreased (despite there being no pharmaceutical industry promotion!). Patients with a classical presentation of bipolar disorder with clear-cut onset and recovery from episodes, and an absence of co-morbid complications, appear to respond better to lithium treatment than do patients with complicating factors. 'Excellent responders' to lithium are patients who experienced full remissions between episodes and no loss of efficacy over time, and who, in contrast to theories of discontinuation-induced refractoriness, after they discontinued lithium experienced no loss of efficacy when they restarted treatment.

Predictors of nonresponse to lithium have been identified as dysphoric mania, rapid cycling, co-morbid medical disorders, polarity sequence, substance abuse, negative family history or frequent prior episodes (Cookson 1997; McIntyre *et al.*, 2001).

Augmentation of antidepressants in resistant depression

The use of lithium as an adjunctive therapy has been suggested for about a decade, and a meta-analysis suggested that the strategy is indeed effective (*Bandolier*, 2000). It is recommended that lithium augmentation of conventional antidepressants should be for at least 7 days and at doses sufficient to reach effective levels of lithium, more than or equal to 0.5 mEq/L.

For reviews see NICE (2004) Clinical Guideline 23, Baldessarini and Tondo (2000), Burgess *et al.* (2003), McIntyre *et al.* (2001), *Bandolier* (2000), *Journal of Clinical Psychiatry* supplement 9 (2000). It is important to realise that much resistant depression responding to lithium is actually undiagnosed bipolar disorder.

Pharmacokinetic profile (ADME)

Lithium is administered orally as the carbonate (solid) or citrate (liquid) form.

Table 9.2 Oral lithium preparations available in the UK

Salt	Preparation	Formulation[a]	Lithium content (mmol or mEq)	Manufacturer
Lithium carbonate	Camcolit	250 mg f/c	6.8	Norgine
		400 mg m/r f/c	10.8	
	Lithonate	400 mg m/r f/c	10.8	TEVA UK
	Liskonum	450 mg m/r f/c	12.2	GSK
	Priadel	200 mg m/r	5.4	Sanofi-Aventis
		400 mg m/r	10.8	
Lithium citrate	Li-liquid	509 mg/5 mL	5.4 per 5 mL (yellow)	Rosemont
	Li-liquid	1018 mg/5 mL	10.8 per 5 mL (orange)	
	Priadel liquid	520 mg/5 mL	5.4 per 5 mL	Sanofi-Aventis

Source: BNF No. 49, March 2005.

[a] f/c, film coated; m/r, modified release.

Lithium preparations available in the UK

Table 9.2 lists lithium preparations available in the UK. Preparations vary in bioavailability and release characteristics (see Figure 9.1). In clinical practice this may be of limited importance, though some authors believe that changing the preparation should carry the same precautions as initiating lithium. Camcolit and Lithonate (Table 9.2) are the same formulation. There is no evidence that one formulation is more effective than another, but they are not bioequivalent, with differences in bioavailability, rate of absorption and serum concentrations.

Lithium Chloride Injection 0.15 mmol/mL (Marketing Authorisation holder LiDCo Ltd) is used as a diagnostic tool for testing cardiac output. This procedure is not suitable for patients who are already taking lithium.

N.B. 200 mg lithium carbonate is approximately equivalent to 509 mg lithium citrate, equivalent to 5.4 mmol of lithium.

Lithium is available as Serenity (lithium orotate containing 4.6 mg elemental lithium per tablet of 120 mg) available via the Internet 'without the need for blood monitoring'. The use of such products should not be supported.

Absorption

The first absorption half-life of lithium liquid is about 9 min where the dose is immediately distributed into a smaller central compartment

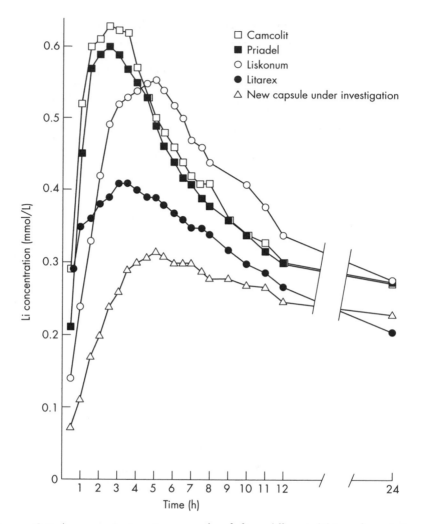

Figure 9.1 A concentration–time graph of five different lithium formulations. Reproduced with permission of Lippincott, Williams & Wilkins from Shelley and Silverstone (1986).

consisting of 20–40% of the body weight. The bioavailability of lithium is 100% for normal-release preparations and between 60% and 90% for modified-release products.

When the pharmacokinetics of solid lithium preparations has been compared with liquid lithium citrate preparations, the results show that whereas the 12 h steady-state levels are similar, there are significant differences in the rate of absorption between the formulations (Markar and Ascough, 1991).

The main differences between the liquid and solid forms is that lithium citrate is absorbed more quickly than lithium carbonate modified-release preparations and the area under the curve from 0 to 5 h is significantly higher for the liquid than for tablets. Modified-release preparations are designed to minimise nausea and tremor.

The manufacturers of Priadel liquid recommend that it be given in two divided doses to avoid high peak lithium levels; however, this increases renal damage compared to once-daily dosing. Once the maintenance dose has reached steady state, 12-h serum concentrations of lithium given twice daily are similar to those on standard-release oral tablets. There is no significant difference in the release characteristics of Priadel and Camcolit.

Lithium absorption throughout the alimentary canal can produce problems at the absorption stage and in the large intestine. Ideally there should be complete distribution of lithium released from the formulation so that no unabsorbed lithium reaches the large intestine to be reabsorbed, attracting water and causing troublesome diarrhoea. Further problems can arise as bioavailability is also affected by diarrhoea, with sodium being lost in the loose stools.

Figure 9.2 shows areas of the alimentary canal involved in lithium absorption.

Distribution

Lithium volume of distribution, $V_d = 0.7 \, L/kg$ (0.42 L/kg in obese adults).

Lithium concentrations in the serum follow an open two-compartment model with the first absorption into the central compartment. The 12-h standardised lithium measurement is usually 12–18 h post dose, after distribution is complete.

After absorption (see Figure 9.3) there is a slower distribution or alpha phase to the rest of the body with a half-life of approximately 6 h, and with an initial volume of distribution of 0.25–0.3 L/kg. This eventually reaches an apparent total distribution volume of 50–120% of the body weight with a half-life of 18 h and final apparent volume of distribution of approximately 0.7–1.0 L/kg. Although this volume of distribution is approximately equal to that of body water, lithium concentrates in various intracompartmental spaces and equilibrates very slowly with the extracellular fluid. Half-life also increases with repeated dosing and after one year can increase by a factor of 1.29–1.4.

At steady state, different tissues have markedly different concentrations of lithium. Lithium concentrations in the systemic circulation

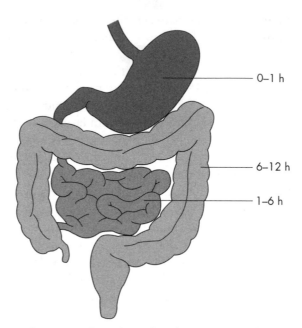

Figure 9.2 Lithium absorption throughout the alimentary canal: 0–1 h Stomach: nausea and tremor associated with rapid absorption of lithium; 1–6 h Small intestine: usually a trouble-free area; 6–12 h Large intestine: lithium not absorbed attracts water and causes loose stools.

are approximately twice those found in red blood cells, muscle and cerebrospinal fluid and similar to those found in the heart and lung. Higher concentrations than in plasma are found in saliva, brain, thyroid gland and bone (Ward *et al.*, 1994).

Elimination

Lithium is eliminated almost exclusively via the renal route; negligible amounts are lost through the faeces and sweat. Lithium is filtered by the kidneys with 80% reabsorbed. Renal tubular reabsorption of lithium is closely linked with sodium reabsorption and is influenced by changes in the renal clearance of sodium. In patients with a normal sodium balance, lithium clearance is approximately 25% creatinine clearance. However, a number of factors influence lithium clearance, the most important being renal function and sodium balance.

Lithium clearance has been reported to be accelerated in acute mania, when patients may require up to 50% more of their usual maintenance dose.

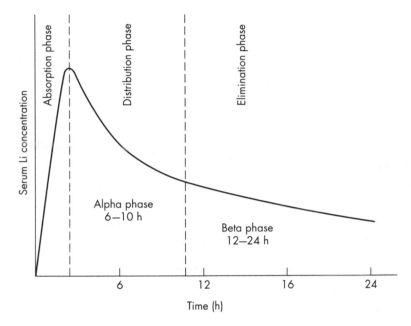

Figure 9.3 Lithium concentrations in serum following a single dose.

Lithium in pregnancy

Lithium is an established teratogen, classified by the FDA as Category D (evidence of human fetal risk, but benefits to the pregnant woman may outweigh the risk). Women are advised not to continue taking it during pregnancy. However, the risk to mother and child of relapse of illness has to be weighed against harm to the fetus. Discontinuing lithium should ideally be gradual over weeks or months, as stopping lithium suddenly increases the incidence of relapse (to 50% during pregnancy, or ten times that which would be expected), psychiatric hospitalisation, suicide and greater use of emergency services. The teratogenic effect occurs over the first few weeks, so stopping once pregnancy is confirmed is too late anyway. For a review of managing lithium therapy during pregnancy, see Bazire (2002).

Pharmacokinetics in lithium toxicity

Toxicity does not necessarily correlate with the measured lithium level because toxicity is affected by the nature and type of the poisoning. These can be subdivided into:

- Acute poisoning – voluntary or accidental ingestion in a previously untreated or discontinued patient

- Acute-on-chronic – voluntary or accidental ingestion in a patient currently using lithium
- Chronic or therapeutic poisoning – progressive lithium toxicity, generally in a patient on lithium therapy

An accurate medication list is important because many drugs (e.g., nonsteroidal anti-inflammatory drugs (NSAIDs), diuretics, tetracyclines, phenytoin and ciclosporin) increase lithium toxicity at therapeutic levels.

The extent of the laboratory work-up depends upon the degree of toxicity suspected and other diagnoses under consideration. One should measure serum lithium concentration if any degree of toxicity is suspected; however, keep in mind that suspicion of toxicity should be high in any patient with known lithium use because early toxic symptoms are very vague and nonspecific.

A second serum lithium level measurement 2 h after the first may disclose any trend, bearing in mind that sustained-release lithium preparations take several hours to reach peak concentrations. See Figure 9.4.

In intentional overdoses, co-ingestions are common and a toxicology screen is indicated. Urea, electrolyte and creatinine measurements are important for determining the patient's ability to excrete lithium. Electrolyte disturbances, particularly hyponatraemia, may predispose an individual to lithium toxicity. On an electrocardiogram (ECG), chronic lithium toxicity is frequently associated with depressed ST segments and T-wave inversion with no symptoms or significant sequelae.

Lithium intoxication may result in dysrhythmias, including complete heart block.

Serious cardiac toxicity is uncommon and generally only occurs in individuals with underlying heart disease.

Population data

Lithium salts:
Therapeutic range: Li^+ 0.4–1.2 mmol/L
Lithium carbonate 200 mg is equivalent to 5.4 mmol Li^+
Bioavailability $(F) = 1$
Lithium clearance CL_{Li} (mL/min) $= 0.25$ creatinine clearance (mL/min)
Volume of distribution $V_d = 0.7$ L/kg (0.42 L/kg in the obese)
Alpha phase half life $= 6$ h
Beta phase half life $= 18$ h (24 h with prolonged therapy)

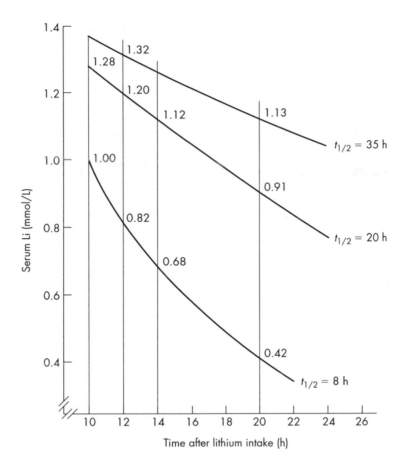

Figure 9.4 Computer-simulated serum lithium concentrations during an interposed day off lithium in three patients, showing characteristic biological half-lives. Reproduced with permission of Lippincott, Williams & Wilkins from Evans, Jusko and Schentag (1992) Lithium in *Applied Pharmacokinetics*, 2nd edn.

Equation resource and examples

To estimate *creatinine clearance* (CL_{cr}) using a recent serum creatinine, the Cockcroft and Gault (1976) equation may be used:

$$CL_{cr} \text{ (mL/min)} = \frac{F \times (140 - \text{Age}) \times \text{Weight (kg)}}{\text{Serum creatinine } (\mu\text{mol/L})} \qquad (9.1)$$

where $F = 1.04$ for females and 1.23 for males.
N.B. This calculation has limitations in some patient groups, for example those who are obese, elderly, emaciated or oedematous.

Lithium clearance, is approximately 25% of creatinine clearance:

$$CL_{Li} = 0.25 \times CL_{cr} \tag{9.2}$$

To calculate the *maintenance dose of lithium* by its elemental content, assuming a one-compartment model and 100% bioavailability:

1 mg lithium carbonate ≡ 0.0271 mmol (or mEq) elemental lithium

1 mg lithium citrate ≡ 0.010 385 mmol (or mEq) elemental lithium

Therefore, 520 mg lithium citrate = (0.010 385 × 520) = 5.4 mmol elemental lithium is equivalent to 200 mg lithium carbonate = (0.0271 × 200) = 5.42 mmol elemental lithium.

To estimate *lithium serum concentration 12 h post dose at steady state* (C_p^{ss}) from a maintenance dose and serum creatinine, the following equation may be used:

$$C_p^{ss} = \frac{F \times MD}{\tau \times CL_{Li}} \tag{9.3}$$

where F = bioavailability = 1 assuming 100%; MD = maintenance dose (in mEq or mmol elemental lithium); τ = dosing interval (h); and CL_{Li} = lithium clearance (L/h).

Example 9.1

Calculate the expected lithium serum concentration for a 40-year-old woman weighing 60 kg, on a maintenance dose of 600 mg Priadel at night, whose recent serum creatinine was 90 μmol/L.

Calculate the expected lithium clearance from creatinine clearance, using equation (9.1):

$$\text{Expected } CL_{cr} \text{ (mL/min)} = \frac{1.04 \times (140 - 40) \times 60}{90}$$
$$= 69.3 \text{ mL/min}$$
$$= (69.3 \times 0.06) \text{ L/h}$$
$$= 4.16 \text{ L/h}$$

Then from equation (9.2):

$$CL_{Li} = 0.25 \times CL_{cr}$$
$$= 0.25 \times 4.16$$
$$= 1.04 \text{ L/h}$$

Each 200 mg Priadel tablet contains approximately 5.4 mmol lithium, so 600 mg Priadel = 16.2 mmol lithium (salt factor accounted for) or $(600 \times 0.0271) = 16.2$ mmol.

Calculate the expected lithium serum concentration using equation (9.3):

$$C_p^{ss} = \frac{F \times MD}{\tau \times CL_{Li}}$$

$$C_p^{ss} = \frac{1 \times 16.2}{24 \times 1.04}$$

$$= 0.65 \text{ mmol/L}$$

There are often individual variations from the expected lithium serum concentration. These calculations should only be used as a guide. Lithium follows first-order kinetics: doubling the dose doubles the serum concentration.

To predict a new dose of lithium carbonate to be taken 12-hourly from previous serum creatinine for the same person:

$$\text{Dose of lithium carbonate} = \frac{C_p^{ss} \times \tau \times CL_{Li}}{S} \qquad (9.4)$$

where C_p^{ss} = steady-state 12-h serum lithium (mmol/L); τ = dosing interval (h); S = salt factor (0.0271 for lithium carbonate); and CL_{Li} = lithium clearance (L/h).

Dosage prediction from a single measurement

Various formulae have been devised to predict lithium dosage from a single serum concentration measurement, thus enabling a suitable steady-state serum concentration to be estimated more quickly. One study compared predictive and empirical lithium dosing versus patient outcome (Marken *et al.*, 1994). The data did not suggest that patient outcome is improved by predictive dosing, but the suggestion of a shorter stay in hospital merits further evaluation.

A procedure suggested by Peet and Pratt (1993) is to start with a daily dosage of 400–600 mg, measure the 12 h serum concentration after 5–7 days, and adjust the dosage according to the result, taking into consideration that steady-state serum concentration is directly proportional to the dosage.

The starting dosage should be lower in the elderly and in patients with clinically relevant physical disorders such as renal impairment or interacting drugs.

If, in acute mania, the serum concentration measured is lower than expected and compliance is assured, it may be that clearance has been accelerated by the manic state.

Example 9.2

A man, 72 kg, age 29 years, serum creatinine 101 μmol/L, who takes 300 mg Priadel 12-hourly, normally has a serum lithium concentration in the therapeutic range. On the last measurement it was 0.3 mmol/L 12 h post dose.

Equations (9.1) and (9.2) will estimate lithium clearance:

$$CL_{Li} = 0.25 \times CL_{cr} = 1.46 \, L/h$$

Substitute present dose of lithium carbonate to estimate the expected lithium serum concentration using equation (9.3):

Predicted serum concentration from 300 mg 12-hourly

$$= \frac{0.0271 \times 300}{12 \times 1.46}$$
$$= 0.464 \, mmol/L$$

His new serum concentration is 0.3 mmol/L.

His lithium clearance has changed during a manic phase. To estimate the present lithium clearance for dose adjustment (equation 9.4):

$$\text{Dose of lithium carbonate (mg)} = \frac{C_p^{ss} \, (mmol/L) \times \tau \, (h) \times CL_{Li} \, (L/h)}{S}$$

$$300 = \frac{0.3 \times 12 \, CL_{Li}}{0.0271}$$

$$CL_{Li} = \frac{300 \times 0.0271}{0.3 \times 12}$$
$$= 2.26 \, L/h$$

Substitute the new clearance into equation (9.4) to estimate a dose that will give a serum concentration of 0.8 mmol/L:

$$\text{Dose of lithium carbonate (mg)} = \frac{C_p^{ss} \, (mmol/L) \times \tau \, (h) \times CL_{Li} \, (L/h)}{S}$$

$$\text{Dose} = \frac{0.8 \times 12 \times 2.26}{0.0271}$$
$$= 800 \, mg \, \text{12-hourly}$$

Reason for request

Routine lithium monitoring every 2–6 months is a requirement during maintenance treatment to minimise the risk of toxicity, along with thyroid function and renal function including 6-monthly serum calcium. Many negligence claims have incurred costs for lack of regular lithium monitoring and interactions with other prescribed drugs (Nicholson and Fitzmaurice, 2002), especially co-prescribed NSAIDs.

Monitoring patients on lithium is not a complex technical task, but communication gaps, lack of clear lines of responsibility and organisation, and different approaches to monitoring perpetuate the ongoing problems. The development of lithium or mood disorder clinics and the application of instant lithium analysers improve patient and healthcare professional involvement.

Factors affecting therapeutic range including important drug interactions

Dosing frequency

Higher 12-h serum concentrations and lower peaks can be expected from more frequent dosing. Renal damage is reported to be higher with multiple daily dosing since, although damage is greater with higher peak levels, the kidney has an opportunity to repair itself during the troughs, something denied during steady but higher levels.

Figure 9.5 is a computer-simulated graph showing the variation in 12-h lithium concentrations depending on the dosing schedule.

Drug interactions

Various factors during therapy can seriously affect lithium serum concentrations. More frequent monitoring is necessary when the situations shown in Table 9.3 arise. Combination of two of these factors in the same group, such as NSAIDs plus increasing age, increases the serum concentration further.

Cases of neurotoxicity and increased incidence of extrapyramidal effects have been reported with some drug interactions by various proposed mechanisms. These include certain antipsychotics (haloperidol, phenothiazines), carbamazepine, calcium channel blockers and selective serotonin reuptake inhibitors (SSRIs). Studies attempting to demonstrate

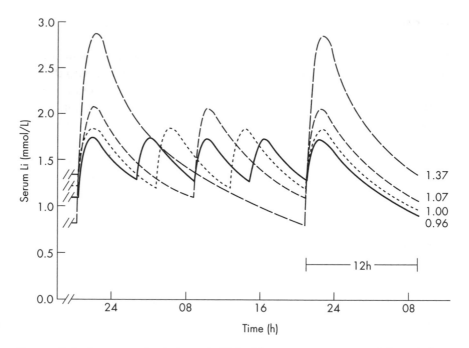

Figure 9.5 Computer-simulation of 12-h lithium concentration. Adapted from *Applied Pharmacokinetics*, 2nd edn, Lippincott Williams & Wilkins.

this effect have had differing results, so it appears to be due to individual sensitivity.

Drug–herb interactions

Herbs that have a diuretic component have the potential to increase the risk of toxicity with lithium. These include agrimony, artichoke, boldo, broom, buchu, burdock, celery, cornsilk, couchgrass, dandelion, devil's claw, elder, guaiacum, java tea, juniper, nettle, pokeroot, shepherd's purse, squill, uva ursi (bearberry) and yarrow.

Changes in renal function

Because lithium is eliminated almost exclusively by the kidneys, renal dysfunction is the most important disorder that affects lithium pharmacokinetics. The clearance rate of lithium decreases in proportion to creatinine clearance. In adults, the ratio of lithium clearance to creatinine

Table 9.3 Factors reported to affect lithium serum concentration

Lower	Variable or no effect	Raise
Acetazolamide	Amiloride	ACE inhibitors – not clinically important in every patient[a]
Aminophylline	Angiotensin II antagonists	Chronic lithium
Caffeine large amount	Aspirin	Metronidazole
Ispaghula husk/Psyllium	Furosemide	Methyldopa (case reports)
Pregnancy[b]	Sulindac	Most NSAIDs[c]
Sodium supplementation	Paracetamol	Thiazide diuretics
Effervescent preparations		Dehydration/volume depletion/diarrhoea
OTC antacids or urinary alkalinisers		Renal impairment
		Sodium loss
		Increasing age

[a] ACE inhibitors important if used in patients of advanced age, with congestive heart failure or renal insufficiency or with volume depletion.
[b] Lithium clearance and serum concentrations return to prepregnancy values after delivery.
[c] NSAIDs = nonsteroidal anti-inflammatory drugs (sulindac excluded, very few reports of raised lithium). It is suggested that NSAIDs inhibit the synthesis of the renal prostaglandin PGE_2 so that renal blood flow is reduced, thereby reducing the renal excretion of lithium.

clearance is 20–25%, but in a manic episode this rises to about 30%. Because of the decrease in clearance in patients with renal failure, the half-life of lithium increases to about 40–50 h.

Renal clearance of lithium is influenced by the state of sodium balance and fluid hydration. Lithium is reabsorbed by the proximal tubule by the same mechanisms that maintain sodium balance.

Lifestyle factors

Patients must be warned of any factor that causes sodium depletion such as diarrhoea and excessive perspiration. Adjustment of the lithium dose to compensate for strenuous exercise, hot climates, use of saunas or alcohol consumption is not usually required, but there is no substitute for patient education regarding salt and fluid replacement and signs of impending toxicity. The best advice to patients is not to ignore feelings of thirst, to avoid overuse of caffeine and alcohol, and to maintain adequate fluid intake at all times (2.5–3 L/day).

Clinical case studies

CASE STUDY 9.1

R.H. is 36-year-old man (inpatient) diagnosed with bipolar affective disorder with aggressive tendencies. He was prescribed Priadel 1200 mg nocte; serum concentration at steady state, 0.9 mmol/L. After a few weeks he was observed palming the tablets (confirmed by follow-up serum concentration <0.2 mmol/L). To ensure adherence, the formulation was changed to Priadel liquid, 1527 mg nocte (15 mL). R.H. remained in hospital another two weeks being verbally aggressive to other patients and staff. Adherence to the liquid formulation was checked every day, and steady-state lithium serum concentration result was 0.38 mmol/L.

How would you explain this?
The wrong equivalent dose was prescribed, or he took a single tablet 3–4 h before being tested.

What dose of lithium citrate would you advise as the nearest equivalent to 1200 mg lithium carbonate?
Bioequivalence of Priadel tablets to Priadel liquid:
509 mg lithium citrate is approximately equivalent to 200 mg lithium carbonate

> Priadel liquid contains 509 mg lithium citrate in 5 mL
> 1200 mg lithium carbonate = 6 × 200 mg

Therefore, the correct nearest equivalent dosage would be 6 × 5 mL spoonfuls = 30 mL Priadel liquid.

CASE STUDY 9.2

A.R. is a 54-year-old woman (weight 51.8 kg, height 165 cm) with resistant depression. She has been taking lithium for many years. Her presenting complaint is a coarse tremor, persistent diarrhoea (for which she purchases loperamide capsules), and recent weight loss. Her current treatment is lofepramine 70 mg t.d.s. and Priadel 400 mg nocte.

She was so troubled by diarrhoea that her GP referred her for investigations for irritable bowel syndrome. These proved inconclusive.

→

⟩ **CASE STUDY 9.2** (continued)

She has a noticeable suntan. Concordance with medication is good.
Lithium serum concentrations 12–14 h post dose:

10/11/01   0.79 mmol/L
09/02/03   0.76 mmol/L
04/05/03   1.67 mmol/L

On comments about the suntan and weight loss, she tells you that she has bought herself a sun bed, which she has been using most nights for the last few months. The secret of the weight loss is a herbal preparation containing uva ursi, bearberry, buchu and juniper.

What advice and investigations would you need for Mrs A.R.?

Check the timing of the blood taken – it may be after a morning dose.

Heavy perspiration without fluid replacement can lead to sodium loss, increasing the risk of raised lithium concentration. This can precipitate diarrhoea, a sign of toxicity. Chronic diarrhoea is a common complaint without other signs of toxicity, but the increased fluid loss could exacerbate this further if allowed to continue.

As lithium levels were constant before the sun bed use, excessive perspiration could have raised levels. Check also for over-the-counter and herbal remedies purchased.

The sustained-release formulation of lithium can also leave unabsorbed lithium in the colon, causing osmotic watery diarrhoea. Check renal function and urea and electrolytes.

Stop lithium for two days, and measure serum concentration to estimate half-life.

Lithium concentration decay over 48 h was from 1.67 to 0.4 mmol/L. Assuming $t_{1/2} = 24$ h, lithium would decay by a half on the first day to 1.67/2, then by another half on the second day to 0.85/2 = 0.425 mmol/L) (renal function appears stable).

Patient education is vital for patients taking lithium. Written information is not always read. A videotaped lecture explaining lithium preparations (available on loan from Sanofi-Aventis at time of writing) is useful for patients whose concentration is not good enough or who are unable to read leaflets. This should be a requirement for all patients starting lithium. Lithium treatment cards and 'Understanding Priadel' cards are also available from NPA, Local Mental Health Care Trusts and Sanofi-Aventis.

Mrs A.R.'s serum creatinine is 73 μmol/L (30/3/03) (range 40–100 μmol/L (females)). Your advice to stop the lithium for two days and retest is followed and the subsequent serum concentration is 0.4 mmol/L.

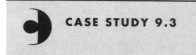

CASE STUDY 9.3

Mrs B., 49 years old, is looking after her husband who has a serious illness. Her lithium serum concentrations are around 0.4 mmol/L. She takes Camcolit 250 mg at night and 125 mg in the morning. She is not sleeping very well and has started to vacuum the carpets at 3 o' clock in the morning.

The last blood test for lithium was 0.29 mmol/L. The severity of her mania and depression in the past required a hospital admission.

What is happening?

Mrs B. is under stress, with traumatic life events, and is showing signs of an impending episode of mania. She may be clearing lithium faster than usual. Concordance with lithium is good, but an increase in dose is indicated urgently at this stage.

What dose of lithium would you recommend?

Calculate the required lithium dose using her last measurement: 0.29 mmol/L.

First calculate her present lithium clearance. The present dose of Camcolit, 125 mg a.m. and 250 mg p.m., averages 187.5 mg per 12 h. The salt factor for lithium carbonate is 0.0271.

$$\text{Measured serum lithium} = \frac{0.0271 \times 187.5}{12 \times \text{Lithium clearance}}$$

$$= 0.29 \, \text{mmol/L}$$

$$\text{Lithium clearance (L/h)} = \frac{0.0271 \times 187.5}{12 \times 0.29}$$

$$= 1.46 \, \text{L/h}$$

If the dose is increased to Camcolit 250 mg twice daily:

$$\text{Predicted lithium serum concentration} = \frac{250 \times 0.0271}{12 \times 1.46}$$

$$= \frac{6.775}{17.52} = 0.39 \, \text{mmol/L}$$

This would not be expected to control an episode of mania, and 500 mg twice daily might be more appropriate. Doubling serum concentrations to dose adjustment would be expected to give a serum lithium concentration of $0.39 \times 2 = 0.77 \, \text{mmol/L}$.

CASE STUDY 9.4

Patient O.W. is a 27-year old woman treated for bipolar depression with lithium and moclobemide. She attends the lithium clinic in tears, saying that 'Everything is hopeless'. She is in a lot of pain, has put on over 10 kg in weight in the last year, and is constipated. She feels her treatment is not working even though she takes it without fail. She is taking 'Solpadol' (co-codamol 30/500) for pain because she knows of the dangers of using nonsteroidal anti-inflammatory drugs.

Her last lithium serum concentration was low (0.3 mmol/L). Previous results have been between 0.6 and 0.7 mmol/L.

What further information do you need?
The constipation is being treated with 'Andrew's liver salts', 1–2 teaspoons a day.

What explanations can you give her for the low lithium?
The constipation is probably caused by the codeine in Solpadol. The combination of the extra sodium in the effervescent preparations has decreased her lithium serum concentration. Advise her to take them in tablet form. Weight gain should be managed, avoiding drastic changes in salt intake and water intake.

References/Further reading

Amdisen A, Carson S W (1992). Lithium clinical pharmacokinetics. In: Evans W E, Schentag J J, Jerome J, eds. *Applied Pharmacokinetics*, 3rd edn. Spokane: Applied Therapeutics.

Anon (1999). Using lithium safely. *Drug Ther Bull* 37: 22–24.

Baldessarini R J, Tondo L (2000). Does lithium treatment still work? Evidence of stable responses over three decades. *Arch Gen Psychiatry* 57(2): 187–190.

Bandolier (2000). Lithium augmentation for treatment-resistant depression. *Bandolier* 77(3) http://www.jr2.ox.ac.uk/bandolier/band77/b77-3.html (accessed 16/04/2003).

Bazire S (2002). Lithium prophylaxis, withdrawal and use in pregnancy. In: Taylor D, Lader M, eds. *Case Studies in Psychopharmacology: The Use of Drugs in Psychiatry*, 2nd edn. London: Martin Dunitz.

Birch N J et al. (1993). Lithium prophylaxis: proposed guidelines for good clinical practice. *Lithium* 4: 225–230.

Burgess S et al. (2003). Lithium for maintenance treatment of mood disorders. *Cochrane review*, Issue 1: http://www.cochrane.org/cochrane/revabstr/ab003013.htm (accessed 13/04/2003).

Cockcroft D W, Gault M H (1976). Prediction of creatinine clearance from serum creatinine. *Nephron* 16: 31–41.

Cookson J (1997). Lithium: balancing risks and benefits. *Br J Psychiatry* 171: 120–124.

Fraser K, Martin M, Hunter R et al. (2001). Mood disorders: bipolar conditions. *Pharm J* 266: 824–832.

Goodwin G M (2003). Evidence-based guidelines for treating bipolar disorder: recommendations from the British Association for Psychopharmacology. *J Psychopharmacol* 17(2): 149–173.

Lenox R H, Hahn C G (2000). Overview of the mechanism of lithium in the brain: fifty-year update. *J Clin Psychiatry* 61 (Suppl. 9): 5–15.

Markar H R, Ascough G (1991). Solid versus liquid lithum – a pharmacokinetic study. *J Clin Pharm Ther* 16: 41–44.

Marken P A, McCrary K E, Lacomb S, et al. (1994). Preliminary comparison of predictive and empiric lithium dosing: impact on patient outcome. *Ann Pharmacother* 10: 1148–1152.

McIntyre R S, Mancini D A, Parikh S, et al. (2001). Lithium revisited. *Can J Psychiatry* 46: 322–327.

NICE (2004). http://www.nice.org.uk (accessed 23/01/2005).

Nicholson J, Fitzmaurice B (2002). Monitoring patients on lithium – a good practice guideline. *Psychiatr Bull* 26: 348–351.

Peet M, Pratt J P (1993). Lithium–current status in psychiatric disorders. *Drugs* 46(1): 7–17.

Sachs G S, Printz D J, Kahn D A, et al. (2000). *Medication Treatment of Bipolar Disorder 2000* (Postgraduate Medicine: The Expert Consensus Guideline Series), 1–104.

Shelley, R K, Silverstone T (1986). Single dose pharmacokinetics of 5 formulations of lithium: a controlled comparison in healthy subjects. *Int Clin Psychopharmacol* 1: 324–331.

Ward M E, Musa M N, Bailey L (1994). Clinical pharmacokinetics of lithium. *J Clin Pharmacol* 34: 280–285.

Winter M E (1996). *Basic Clinical Pharmacokinetics*, 3rd edn. Vancouver: Applied Therapeutics.

Supplements

'Achieving Success in the Management of Bipolar Disorder: Is Lithium Sufficient?' *Journal of Clinical Psychiatry* (2003) 64 (Supplement 5).

'Fifty Years of Lithium Use in the Treatment of Bipolar Disorder'. *Journal of Clinical Psychiatry* (2000) 61 (Supplement 9).

'Lithium in the Treatment of Manic Depressive Illness: An Update'. *Journal of Clinical Psychiatry* (1998) 59 (Supplement 6).

10

Antiepileptics

Ian Chi Kei Wong

Aims and learning outcomes

A trainee health professional with partial seizure walked into the epilepsy clinic; the consultant smiled and asked 'Have you had any more fits?' She replied 'Only once since last time I saw you.' The consultant took out the TDM report. The report showed the plasma level of carbamazepine was ... zero.

As a research pharmacist in a tertiary epilepsy referral centre, I witnessed the above scene personally; obviously this carbamazepine result was extremely important and it confirmed the consultant's suspicion. However, I have also seen many unnecessary TDM reports of antiepileptic drugs ordered; even worse is that some inexperienced clinicians would change patients' treatment based on the wrong interpretation of the drug plasma level.

The purpose of this chapter, is to help you to understand the principle of therapeutic drug monitoring (TDM) in the treatment of epilepsy and to be able to apply it in clinical situations.

After reading this chapter you will be able to:

- Define and classify seizures.
- Describe the basic pharmacological actions of antiepileptic drugs.
- Apply the principles of TDM in the treatment of epilepsy.

Epilepsy and seizures

The epilepsies are among the most common of neurological disorders. Prevalence is approximately 5 per 1000 and, based on this figure, there are 250 000 people in the UK who suffer from epilepsy. Approximately 70% of patients with epilepsy are well controlled by monotherapy with currently available antiepileptic drugs. Another 5–10% of patients are stabilised by the addition of another antiepileptic drug, but there remain over 20% of patients whose seizures are not controlled.

Definition of epilepsy and seizures

Although there has been major advance in the understanding of both the causes and treatments of seizures, the definition has not been changed since 1870. Hughings Jackson defined a seizure in physiological terms as 'a recurrent, disorderly discharge of nerve tissue'. This is still widely accepted and used by leading epileptologists.

On the other hand, epilepsy was defined as 'a chronic disorder characterised by recurrent seizures'. The word *recurrent* is crucial, since a single isolated seizure is not classified as epilepsy.

Epilepsy is not a diagnosis in itself but is a consequence of a wide variety of cerebral diseases. Seizures can occur in response to practically any generalised metabolic disturbance or cerebral pathology. Therefore, it is important for clinicians to identify any possible underlying cause such as alcohol misuse or cerebral tumour.

Classifications of epileptic seizures and syndromes

The type of seizure is an essential factor in determining the treatment. A common reason for the failure of treatment is the misclassification of seizure; for example, ethosuximide is as effective as sodium valproate in the treatment of absence seizures but is ineffective in complex partial seizures. Loss of consciousness is the main feature in both types of seizures, so misclassification can easily arise. In conclusion, it is essential for clinicians and pharmacists to understand the classification of epileptic seizures.

Classification of epileptic seizures

The simplified classification is shown in Box 10.1. There is a fundamental distinction between seizures that arise from a particular area or focus (partial seizures) and those that involve the entire brain at the same time (generalised). Another important feature is the subdivision of partial seizures. When consciousness is impaired during the attack, the partial seizure is classified as complex. When consciousness is preserved, the partial seizure is classified as simple.

Box 10.1 Simplified classification of epileptic seizures

I. **Partial seizures.** (The first clinical and electroencephalographic changes indicate initial activation of a system of neurons limited to part of one cerebral hemisphere.)
   A. Simple partial seizures. (Consciousness is not impaired.)
   B. Complex partial seizures. (Consciousness is impaired; may sometimes begin with simple symptomatology.)
   C. Partial seizures evolving to secondarily generalised seizures.

II. **Generalised seizures.** (The first clinical and electroencephalographic changes indicate initial involvement of both cerebral hemispheres. Motor manifestations are bilateral. The ictal electroencephalographic patterns initially are bilateral, and presumably reflect neuronal discharge which is widespread in both hemispheres.)
   A. Tonic-clonic
   B. Absence
   C. Myoclonic
   D. Tonic
   E. Clonic
   F. Atonic

III. **Unclassified seizures**. (Insufficient data for classification.)

Rationale for therapeutic drug monitoring (TDM)

Some clinicians and pharmacists routinely request TDM in patients taking antiepileptic drugs; however, many of these TDMs are not necessary or are 'unusable'.

Serum level monitoring should only be performed with a clear clinical indication. Indications for monitoring of antiepileptic drug blood levels are (NICE, 2004):

- Detection of nonadherence to the prescribed medication
- Suspected toxicity
- Adjustment of phenytoin dose
- Management of pharmacokinetic interactions
- Specific clinical conditions, for example status epilepticus, organ failure and pregnancy

Drug concentration can only be a guide to optimising dosage. It should not be a sole criterion on which therapeutic decisions are based. Attention must be paid to a patient's clinical situation:

- Side-effects: A patient could have a plasma level within the 'recommended therapeutic range' but experience adverse drug reactions; in this situation dose reduction is warranted.
- Seizure frequency: A patient could have a plasma concentration well below the 'recommended therapeutic range' but with seizures under control; in this situation the patient should remain on the same dose.

Key points to remember when requesting TDM

1. As a pharmacist or clinician, you should be satisfied that there are valid reasons (see above) to request TDM.
2. You should accurately record the following details for the interpretation of the results:
   (a) Patient's details: weight, height, age, sex and type of seizure/epilepsy.
   (b) Treatment:
      (i) Dose of the drug tested.
      (ii) Time of the last dose; most of the drugs should be tested after the absorption phase, and trough concentrations are frequently used.
      (iii) When the drug was initiated or the last dose change, to ensure the plasma level is at a steady state.
      (iv) Concurrent medications that could affect the plasma concentration.
      (v) Concurrent illnesses that could affect the plasma concentration.

Treatment

The treatment for epilepsy is mainly pharmacological, although in selected cases, mainly in patients with a focal lesion in the brain, e.g. hippocampal sclerosis, surgery may be able to cure or reduce the frequency of seizures.

Profiles of antiepileptic drugs

Antiepileptic drugs that may benefit from TDM

Phenytoin

Phenytoin is an effective therapy in generalised tonic-clonic and partial seizures. It was the first-choice treatment for generalised tonic-clonic seizures but it has gradually been replaced by sodium valproate and carbamazepine.

Phenytoin reduces the amplitude of sodium-dependent action potential by increasing the voltage dependency of steady-state inactivation and by reducing the rate of recovery of sodium channels from inactivation. It has been demonstrated that phenytoin can inhibit the binding of $[^3H]$batrachotoxinin (a toxin that binds to sodium channels at a site related to activation of sodium channel ion flux to sodium channels). This provides strong evidence that phenytoin is acting on sodium channels.

Phenytoin is a hepatic enzyme inducer; it therefore exhibits significant pharmacokinetic interaction with other drugs such as oral contraceptive steroids.

Intoxication is characterised by nystagmus, ataxia, lethargy, and possibly a paradoxical increase in seizures. Severe and prolonged intoxication may cause degeneration of cerebellar Purkinje cells.

Phenytoin can cause osteomalacia and hypocalcaemia, which are partly attributable to interference with vitamin D metabolism. Long-term use of phenytoin may impair utilisation of folic acid to result in megaloblastic anaemia. Gingival hyperplasia occurs in approximately 20% of patients, is generally attributable to a disorder of fibroblast activity, and is exacerbated by poor dental hygiene.

Phenytoin may very rarely produce blood dyscrasias, such as agranulocytosis and aplastic anaemia. Skin rash is an indication for immediate withdrawal to avoid rare but serious exfoliative dermatitis, or even Stevens–Johnson syndrome (a severe bullous rash involving two or more mucosal surfaces).

Pharmacokinetic profile

Unlike most drugs, phenytoin does not exhibit linear pharmacokinetics; as the phenytoin dose is increased, the ability of the body to eliminate it will increase initially but will then reach saturation. Hence, any alteration

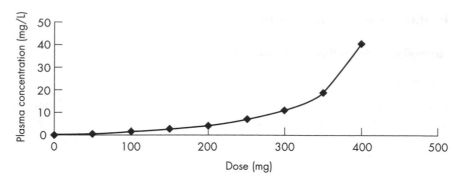

Figure 10.1 Nonlinear pharmacokinetics of phenytoin.

in the metabolism or a small change of dose of phenytoin may result in the loss of seizure control or the precipitation of dose-dependent toxicity (see Figure 10.1).

This type of pharmacokinetic profile has been described as saturable pharmacokinetics, capacity-limited pharmacokinetics, or nonlinear pharmacokinetics. Furthermore, there are large interindividual differences, making dose adjustment challenging, so TDM is particularly useful in phenytoin. The 'usual therapeutic plasma level' has been widely taken as 10–20 mg/L (40–80 μmol/L).

Most of the formulations are as phenytoin sodium salt because this is more soluble and has a more reliable absorption than the phenytoin acid. The excipient may have a significant effect on the absorption: there was an 'outbreak' of phenytoin intoxication after the company changed the excipient from hydrated calcium sulfate to lactose, which caused an unexpected increase in bioavailability.

Phenytoin is rapidly distributed to the body tissues after absorption. Approximately 90% of phenytoin binds to plasma proteins and the percentage of binding is dependent on albumin concentration (only free phenytoin is pharmacologically active). Hypoalbuminaemia will reduce the binding and hence increase the free phenytoin. Bilirubin competes with the same binding sites; therefore, it is necessary to take concurrent illness such as hepatic and renal conditions into consideration.

The majority of phenytoin is metabolised by cytochrome P450 mixed oxidase, and less than 5% of phenytoin is excreted unchanged in the urine.

As phenytoin exhibits saturable pharmacokinetics, its half-life, depending on plasma level, has been cited as between 10 and 40 h.

*Michaelis–Menten equation for the estimation of
plasma concentration*

The rate of change of plasma concentration (V) of a drug such as phenytoin by an enzyme system can be expressed by the Michaelis–Menten equation:

$$V = \frac{V_m \times C_p}{K_m + C_p} \tag{10.1}$$

where V is the rate of metabolism; V_m is the maximum rate of metabolism; K_m is the Michaelis–Menten constant (i.e. drug concentration at which V will be half V_m); and C is the drug concentration.

When equation (10.1) is used in the clinical situation, the daily dose or administration rate of phenytoin (R_a) is substituted for rate of metabolism (V).

R_a = daily dose (R) $\times$ bioavailability factor (F) $\times$ fraction of administered dose that is active drug (S)

The steady-state phenytoin concentration (C_p^{ss}) is substituted for drug concentration (C). The equation can then be derived for steady-state concentrations:

$$R \times F \times S = \frac{V_m \times C_p^{ss}}{K_m + C_p^{ss}} \tag{10.2}$$

$$C_p^{ss} = K_m \frac{R \times F \times S}{V_m - (R \times F \times S)}$$

Use of population data

As practice, use the average population data to demonstrate the effect of dose changing on the plasma level in a 60 kg patient, $V_m = 7$ mg/kg/day, $K_m = 5.7$ mg/L, $F = 1$, $S = 0.92$.

300 mg capsule daily:

$$\begin{aligned}
C_p^{ss}(300\,\text{mg}) &= 5.7[300 \times 1 \times 0.92]/[(7 \times 60) \\
&\quad - (300 \times 1 \times 0.92)] \\
&= 11 \text{ mg/L (lower end of the usual} \\
&\quad \text{therapeutic range)}
\end{aligned}$$

350 mg capsule daily:

$$\begin{aligned}
C_p^{ss}(350\,\text{mg}) &= 5.7[350 \times 1 \times 0.92]/[(7 \times 60) \\
&\quad - (350 \times 1 \times 0.92)] \\
&= 19 \text{ mg/L (higher end of the} \\
&\quad \text{usual therapeutic range)}
\end{aligned}$$

400 mg capsule daily:

$$C_p^{ss}(400\,\text{mg}) = 5.7[400 \times 1 \times 0.92]/[(7 \times 60)$$
$$- (400 \times 1 \times 0.92)]$$
$$= 40\ \text{mg/L (likely to be toxic)}$$

From the above example, it is clear that a small change in the dose could result in a very large change in plasma level.

Population data for estimation of the pharmacokinetic parameters

Population data could be used to estimate the pharmacokinetic parameters. However, as mentioned previously, the intersubject variability is high and it is important to bear in mind that your patient may not be a 'typical' patient to whom the population pharmacokinetics could be applied. Nevertheless, the following have been used:

- $V_m = 7\,\text{mg/kg/day}$.
  For example, a 60-kg patient would give
  $V_m = 7\,\text{mg/kg/day} \times 60\,\text{kg} = 420\,\text{mg/day}$
- K_m: The population K_m is 5.7 mg/L in adults and 5.6–6.6 mg/L in paediatric patients.

Various nomograms have been developed for dose adjustment of phenytoin; the orbit plot (Figure 10.2) is presented here as an example.

Factors affecting therapeutic range

Conditions such as renal and hepatic illness causing hypoalbuminaemia or hyperbilirubinaemia will increase the free phenytoin and it is necessary to measure the free drug instead of the total plasma concentration. Concurrent medications can have significant effects on the phenytoin plasma concentration; refer to Table 10.1 for details.

Fosphenytoin, a prodrug of phenytoin, has been marketed in the UK since 2000. Fosphenytoin has been used for some years in the USA and can be administered intravenously or intramuscularly. Studies have found it to be as effective as phenytoin in treating status epilepticus, with several advantages over its parent drug. Intramuscular administration of fosphenytoin sodium has the benefits of rapid and complete absorption and no requirement for cardiac monitoring. Patients with neurological or neurosurgical disorders that affect consciousness levels, or patients

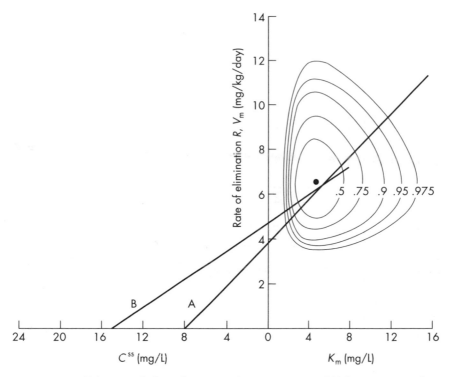

Figure 10.2 Orbit graph for phenytoin dose estimation. With permission from Elsevier Ltd. Walker & Edward (2002). The most probable values of V_m and K_m for a patient may be estimated using a single steady-state phenytoin concentration and a known dosing regimen. The eccentric circles of 'orbits' represent the fraction of the sample patient population whose K_m and V_m values are within that orbit. (1) Plot the daily dose of phenytoin (mg/kg/day) on the vertical line (rate of elimination). (2) Plot the steady-state concentration (C^{ss}) on the horizontal line. (3) Draw a straight line connecting C^{ss} and daily dose through the orbits (line A). (4) The coordinates of the midpoint of the line crossing the innermost orbit through which the line passes are the most probable values for the patient's V_m and K_m. (5) To calculate a new maintenance dose, draw a line from the point determined in step 4 to the new desired C^{ss} (line B). The point at which line B crosses the vertical line (rate of elimination) is the new maintenance dose (mg/kg/day). The line A represents a C^{ss} of 8 mg/L on 276 mg/day of phenytoin acid (300 mg/day of sodium phenytoin) for a 70-kg patient. Line B has been drawn assuming that the new desired steady-state concentration was 15 mg/L (μg/mL). The original figure is modified so that R *and* V_m are in mg/kg/day of phenytoin acid.

for whom the gastrointestinal route is not available, would be well suited to the use of intramuscular fosphenytoin sodium. Side-effects are similar to those of parenteral phenytoin: nystagmus, dizziness, pruritus, paraesthesias, headache, somnolence and ataxia.

Table 10.1 Expected changes in plasma concentrations when an antiepileptic drug (AED) is added to a pre-existing regimen

AED added	Pre-existing AED														
	PB	PHT	PRM	ETS	CBZ	VPA	OXC	LTG	GBP	TPM	TGB	LEV	ZNS	VGB	FBM
PB	..	PHT↑↓	NCCP	ETS⇓	CBZ⇓	VPA⇓	H-OXC⇓	LTG⇓	↔	TPM⇓	TGB⇓	↔	ZNS⇓	↔	FBM⇓
PHT	PB↑	..	PRM↓ PB↑	ETS⇓	CBZ⇓	VPA⇓	H-OXC⇓	LTG⇓	↔	TPM⇓	TGB⇓	↔	ZNS⇓	↔	FBM⇓
PRM	NCCP	PHT↑↓	..	ETS⇓	CBZ⇓	?	?	LTG⇓	↔	TPM⇓	TGB⇓	↔	ZNS⇓	↔	FBM⇓
ETS	↔	NE	NE	..	↔	VPA↓	NE	NE	NE	NE	NE	NE	NE	NE	NE
CBZ	↔	PHT↑↓	PRM↓ PB↑	ETS⇓	..	VPA⇓	H-OXC⇓	LTG⇓	↔	TPM⇓	TGB⇓	↔	ZNS⇓	NE	FBM⇓
VPA	PB⇑	PHT↓*	PB⇑	ETS↑↓	CBZ-E↑	..	::	LTG⇑	↔	TPM↓	↔	↔	↔	NE	↔
OXC	PB↑	PHT↑	?	?	CBZ↓	↔	..	LTG↓	NE	?	NE	NE	?	NE	↔
LTG	↔	↔	NE	NE	↔	↔	NE	..	NE	NE	NE	↔	↔	NE	↔
GBP	↔	↔	NE	NE	↔	↔	NE	NE	..	NE	NE	↔	NE	NE	NE
TPM	↔	PHT↑	↔	NE	↔	VPA↓	?	?	NE	..	::	NE	?	NE	NE
TGB	↔	↔	↔	NE	↔	↔	NE	NE	::	::	..	::	NE	NE	NE
LEV	↔	↔	↔	NE	↔	↔	NE	↔	↔	NE	NE	..	NE	::	NE
ZNS	↔	↔	NE	NE	CBZ↑↓	↔	?	↔	NE	NE	NE	NE	..	NE	NE
VGB	PB↓	PHT↓	PRM↓ PB↓	NE	CBZ↑	↔	NE	NE	NE	NE	NE	NE	::	..	NE
FBM	PB⇑	PHT⇑	?	?	CBZ↓ CBZ-E↑	VPA⇑	↔	↔	NE	?	?	NE	?	↔	..

Reproduced from Patsalos et al. (2003) with permission of Elsevier Ltd.

PB = phenobarbital; PHT = phenytoin; PRM = primidone; ETS = ethosuximide; CBZ = carbamazepine; VPA = valproic acid; OXC = oxcarbazepine; LTG = lamotrigine; GBP = gabapentin; TPM = topiramate; TGB = tiagabine; LEV = levetiracetum; ZNS = zonisamide; VGB = vigabatrin; FBM = felbamate; H-OXC = 10-hydroxyoxcarbazepine (active metabolite of OXC); CBZ-E = carbamazepine-10, 11-epoxide. NE = none expected; *free (pharmacologically active) concentration may increase; NCCP = not commonly coprescribed; ↔ = no change; ↓ = a minor (or inconsistent) decrease in plasma concentration; ⇓ = a clinically significant decrease in plasma concentration; ↑ = a minor (or inconsistent) increase in plasma concentration; ⇑ = a clinically significant increase in plasma concentration.

However, clinicians and pharmacists must bear in mind that the dose of fosphenytoin sodium should be prescribed in terms of phenytoin sodium equivalent (PE):

150 mg fosphenytoin $\equiv$ 100 mg phenytoin sodium

Carbamazepine

Carbamazepine is first-line therapy for patients with localisation-related epilepsy manifesting as partial seizures and secondary generalised tonic-clonic seizure. It has the capability to induce its own metabolism, a property known as autoinduction. Consequently, the initial dose should be low and the dose should be built up gradually over weeks or months, when autoinduction is complete. Like phenytoin, it can induce the metabolism of other drugs such as phenytoin and sodium valproate.

The action of carbamazepine is similar to that of phenytoin. It reduces the frequency of sustained repetitive firing of action potentials in mouse central neuron cell culture. Again similar to phenytoin, carbamazepine has been shown to inhibit the binding of [^{3}H]batrachotoxinin to sodium channels.

Adverse effects include nausea, vomiting, ataxia, drowsiness, headache, diplopia, dizziness and rash. Rarely hepatotoxicity, cardiac conduction disturbances and exfoliative dermatitis may occur. Transient leucopenia occurs in about 10% of patients, usually in the first month of therapy. More substantial persistent leucopenia is rare and responds to discontinuation of carbamazepine. Inappropriate antidiuretic hormone-like action and hyponatraemia is very common, but it does not usually cause clinical problems. There is a substantial increase in the risk of neural tube defects when carbamazepine is administered during pregnancy.

Pharmacokinetics

Absorption of carbamazepine is slow and erratic. There is no intravenous formulation available for absolute bioavailability assessment; the estimated bioavailability is 75–85%.

Carbamazepine distributes to tissues rapidly because it is highly lipid-soluble. Approximately 75–85% of carbamazepine is bound to plasma proteins. The volume of distribution (V_d) is between 0.8 and 2 L/kg.

The main metabolite is carbamazepine-10,11-epoxide, which is then hydrolysed to carbamazepine-10,11-*trans*-dihydrodiol. Less than 2% of the parent drug is excreted unchanged in the urine. Carbamazepine-10, 11-epoxide is pharmacologically active and contributes to the antiepileptic effects as well as the side-effects; it is, therefore, sometimes also useful to monitor the levels of both epoxide and parent drug.

The half-life of a single dose of carbamazepine can be as long as 55 h; however following repeated dosing, the autoinduction process will reduce the half-life to between 5 and 26 h. The average clearance of carbamazepine is 0.133 L/kg/h but clearance is very variable.

Carbamazepine exhibits dose-dependent pharmacokinetics and 4–10 mg/L (15–40 μmol/L) is frequently cited as the targeted therapeutic level for long-term treatment; however, it is more important to adjust dosage according to response rather than according to the plasma level.

Slow-release preparations are widely used to reduce the peak plasma level so that patients are less likely to experience dose-dependent side-effects. The bioavailability of slow-release preparations is lower, so it is important to adjust the dose accordingly. The author has seen some patients develop acute toxicity that required hospitalisation after changing from a slow-release formulation to the same dose of a normal-release formulation.

Factors affecting therapeutic range

The most important factor is autoinduction; dose incrementation is required during the early period of treatment. Carbamazepine is metabolised by the liver, so severe hepatic disease will reduce its rate of metabolism. The metabolism of carbamazepine can be significantly affected by other concurrent antiepileptic medications. See Table 10.1 for more details.

Barbiturates and primidone

Phenobarbital is the major barbiturate used in the treatment of epilepsy. Phenobarbital is effective in the treatment of generalised tonic-clonic and partial seizures, although its general CNS-depressant properties relegate its use to that as a second-line agent.

Although it has been suggested that phenobarbital has a wide-range of activity in experimental models, it is widely accepted that the antiepileptic activity is mainly due to the effect on the GABA receptor. Barbiturates enhance the $GABA_A$ receptor current by binding to an allosteric regulatory site on the receptor. Results from fluctuation analysis suggest that phenobarbital increases the mean channel open duration of $GABA_A$ receptor current without altering channel conductance. Single-channel recordings of barbiturate-enhanced single $GABA_A$ receptor currents directly demonstrate that barbiturates increase the mean time for which the chloride channel is open but do not alter receptor conductance or opening frequency.

Drowsiness, and in children irritability and hyperactivity, are the main adverse effects of phenobarbital, but patients tend to become tolerant to the sedative action. It is a potent inducer of mixed-function oxidases and other hepatic enzymes; it therefore causes significant pharmacokinetic interaction with other drugs such as phenytoin and contraceptive steroids. Phenobarbital is still the main treatment for epilepsy in Third World countries because it is the least expensive antiepileptic treatment, and it is no less effective than the more selective antiepileptic drugs.

Primidone, which is metabolised to phenobarbital and phenylethylmalonamide, probably owes its anticonvulsant properties to these metabolites and has a similar place in the treatment of epilepsy. Primidone was withdrawn from the market in 2003 and most patients have been transferred to other treatment; we will therefore not discuss this preparation further.

Pharmacokinetics

The bioavailability of phenobarbital is between 80% and 100% and peak plasma concentration occurs 1–3 h post oral dose. Absorption can be delayed by the presence of food. Phenobarbital readily distributes into tissues, and the volume of distribution has been reported between 0.6 and 1 L/kg. Protein binding is approximately 50%.

Phenobarbital is partly metabolised and partly excreted unchanged in the urine. The half-life and clearance have been reported as 10–120 h and 0.006–0.009 L/kg/h, respectively.

Phenobarbital exhibits linear pharmacokinetics, but there is considerable variation between patients. A plasma concentration between 10 and 40 mg/L (40–170 µmol/L) has been suggested as a guide to therapy; however, tolerance could occur and make the value of TDM less than for phenytoin and carbamazepine. Concurrent antiepileptic drugs could have significant effects on the plasma level (see Table 10.1).

Antiepileptic drugs that have little evidence to support TDM

Established antiepileptic drugs

Sodium valproate

Sodium valproate has a broad spectrum of antiepileptic activity; it is effective against generalised tonic-clonic seizures, absence seizures, myoclonic seizures in patients with primary generalised epilepsy, partial seizures and secondary generalised tonic-clonic seizures in patients with localisation-related epilepsies. Some clinicians have suggested that the broader spectrum of activity of sodium valproate makes it the drug of choice for use by relatively inexperienced and inexpert clinicians treating epilepsy.

In vitro study suggests that sodium valproate blocks sustained high-frequency repetitive firing of neurons in culture; this effect is similar to that of phenytoin and carbamazepine. However, unlike for phenytoin, biochemical studies have failed to demonstrate an interaction between sodium valproate and Na^+ channels at relevant concentrations.

Because sodium valproate is very effective against absence seizures it has been suggested that it may interact with calcium channels. Animal studies have also suggested that sodium valproate can increase the level of GABA in the whole brain and nerve endings. There is an increase in plasma and CSF levels of GABA in patients being treated with usual clinically effective doses of sodium valproate. Although it has been reported that sodium valproate is a GABA transaminase inhibitor, it failed to produce inhibition *in vivo* or *in vitro* in intact cells. In conclusion, sodium valproate has a wide spectrum of antiepileptic effect, suggesting that its clinical activity may be related to a combination of mechanisms.

Adverse effects of sodium valproate include nausea, tremor, transient hair loss, weight gain and pancreatitis. The most serious side-effect is fatal hepatotoxicity, which occurs mainly in children under 2 years old. Hyperammonaemia and rarely thrombocytopenia have also been reported. There is a substantial increase in the risk of neural tube defects when sodium valproate is administered during pregnancy.

Unlike other major antiepileptic drugs, sodium valproate is a hepatic enzyme inhibitor and displays first-order pharmacokinetics. It can inhibit the metabolism of other drugs and can cause toxicity, notably with lamotrigine-induced rash.

No clear concentration–response relationship has been demonstrated; TDM is therefore generally not useful with sodium valproate.

Benzodiazepines

Clonazepam and clobazam are the benzodiazepines most commonly used. They play a secondary role owing to their sedative and tolerance-inducing properties. Clonazepam is useful for treating myoclonic seizures.

Intravenous or rectal diazepam is indicated for termination of prolonged or repeated seizures.

Benzodiazepines have been shown to have high affinity for a specific binding site (benzodiazepine receptor) on the $GABA_A$ receptor and to potentiate the effects of GABA. The frequency of opening of chloride channels is increased, causing hyperpolarisation and reduction in neuronal firing rate.

Diazepam is highly lipophilic and readily enters the central nervous system. Its duration of action after a single intravenous bolus (for status epilepticus) is relatively short because it rapidly redistributes from the brain to peripheral tissues. Lorazepam undergoes less rapid redistribution from the brain than diazepam and is a longer-acting alternative for control of status epilepticus.

Ethosuximide

Ethosuximide is indicated only for generalised absence seizures. Initial dose is 500 mg/day, increasing to 500–2000 mg/day. Ethosuximide has been shown to affect T-calcium currents in thalamic neurons. The adverse effects are nausea, drowsiness, anorexia and headache. Rare cases of rash, leucopenia and lupus-like syndromes have been reported.

Newer antiepileptic drugs

There are only some prospective data on the serum concentration–effect relationships, and few studies have been designed primarily to study these relationships. As TDM is not widely practised for the newer antiepileptic drugs, there are no generally accepted target ranges for any of these drugs, and for most a wide range in serum concentration is associated with clinical efficacy. Furthermore, a considerable overlap in drug concentrations related to toxicity and nonresponse is reported; as a result, routine monitoring in general cannot be recommended at present. However, Johannessen *et al.* (2003) have suggested some tentative target ranges for some new antiepileptic drugs and readers interested in this topic should refer to that paper.

Below are summarized the key characteristics of some newer antiepileptic drugs as an introduction for the reader. The American Academy of Neurology and the American Epilepsy Society have conducted two comprehensive reviews on the efficacy and tolerability of new antiepileptic drugs in new-onset epilepsy and refractory epilepsy (French, 2004a,b); these two reviews are highly recommended to readers who want to learn more about the new antiepileptic drugs.

Gabapentin

Structural analogues of GABA were synthesised to test antiepileptic effects in animal models. Gabapentin was found to have antiepileptic activity as part of such a programme. It is licensed as add-on therapy for partial seizures and partial seizures with secondary generalisation.

The initial dose of gabapentin is 300 mg daily for the first day, 300 mg twice daily for the second day, 300 mg three times daily for the third day; the maintenance dose is up to 2400 mg/day.

Gabapentin has been shown to block voltage-dependent sodium ion channels and to increase the release of GABA at therapeutically relevant concentrations. Laboratory study has shown that gabapentin binds to a novel site, possibly the neutral L-amino acid transport carrier.

Very few serious adverse drug reactions have been reported; most of those are CNS-related, e.g. drowsiness, dizziness, headache and ataxia. Aggravation of seizures has been reported frequently.

Lamotrigine

It has long been known that some antiepileptic drugs can lower the serum folate levels, and that folate supplementation can worsen seizures. The former Wellcome Research Laboratories looked among a number of recognised antifolate compounds for a new antiepileptic drug. The dosage is very complicated and depends on the concurrent medications. Inappropriate dosages potentially cause hypersensitivity reactions (refer to the British National Formulary for advice).

Lamotrigine has only very mild antifolate activity; the antiepileptic effects of lamotrigine are likely to be due to the inhibition of sodium currents by interaction with the inactivated channel and the inhibitory effects on the release of glutamate.

Lamotrigine is licensed (in the UK) as first-line treatment for partial seizures and secondary generalised tonic clonic seizures and for primary generalised epilepsy. Adverse drug reactions are mainly CNS-related, e.g. ataxia, diplopia, headache, tremor and drowsiness. However, rash and hypersensitivity are major problems and fatal cases have been reported. Lamotrigine also has significant interactions with sodium val-proate and carbamazepine (see Table 10.1).

Levetiracetam

Levetiracetam is an analogue of piracetam but has a broader spectrum of seizure activity. Although the exact mechanism of its action is yet to be defined, various theories have been proposed, including changes in GABA metabolism and turnover, inhibition of depolarising ion currents, calcium channel-dependent effects and dopaminergic activation. The initial dose is 1000 mg/day, increasing to 3000 mg/day.

Levetiracetam is a new antiepileptic drug and the safety profile remains to be established. Somnolence, asthenia, headache and dizziness have been reported. Levetiracetam administered as adjunctive therapy does not appear to interact with other anticonvulsant drugs.

Oxcarbazepine

Oxcarbazepine is the 10-keto analogue of carbamazepine. It is functionally a prodrug activated by liver metabolism. The active metabolite is 10,11-dihydro-10-hydroxy-5*H*-dibenzo(*b,f*)azepine-5-carboxamide.

Oxcarbazepine is less likely to cause hypersensitivity reaction and drug interactions than carbamazepine, while retaining similar efficacy and antiepileptic effects. The initial dosage is 300 mg twice daily and the usual maintenance dose is 600–2400 mg/day.

Piracetam

Piracetam was originally introduced as a 'smart drug' and was subsequently found to be effective in myoclonic seizures. Piracetam increases blood flow at the capillary level, but the drug's antimyoclonic action is unclear. It has a good safety record. The initial dosage is 7.2 g/day in 2–3 divided doses and can be increased to 20 g/day. One tablet contains 800 mg, so a patient can take up to 25 tablets a day.

Tiagabine

Tiagabine is a specific GABA reuptake inhibitor. It has recently been released in several countries as adjunctive therapy in partial seizures. The initial dose is 5 mg twice daily and the maintenance dose is

30–40 mg/day (with enzyme inducer) and 15–30 mg/day (without enzyme inducer).

Tiagabine is a relatively new drug and the safety profile remains to be established. The usual CNS-related adverse drug reaction have been reported; nonconvulsive status epilepticus has been reported in a few patients.

Topiramate

Several mechanisms of action have been postulated for topiramate, including state-dependent sodium channel blockade and enhancement of GABA-mediated chloride influx into neurons. Topiramate also inhibits kainate activity on the kainate/AMPA subtype of glutamate receptors and weakly inhibits carbonic anhydrase.

Topiramate is licensed for use as an adjunctive therapy in partial seizures with or without secondary generalisation. The initial dose is 50 mg at night and the maximum maintenance dose is 800 mg/day. This is a relatively new drug and the safety profile remains to be established. Adverse drug reactions are mainly CNS-related, e.g. drowsiness, dizziness, headache, ataxia and neuropsychiatric adverse drug reactions. Other adverse drug reactions are weight loss and formation of kidney stones (renal calculi).

Vigabatrin

The synthesis of vigabatrin represents an advance in drug design. It was modelled on the structure of the neurotransmitter GABA and the traditional 'search for a needle in the haystack' by the screening of hundreds of molecules was replaced by a systematic 'drug design' approach. The initial dose is 1 g/day, and the maximum dose is 3 g/day.

The main antiepileptic effect of vigabatrin is due to inhibition of GABA transaminase. The inhibition of glutamate and aspartate synthesis and of GABA uptake may also contribute to the antiepileptic effect.

Vigabatrin is licensed for the treatment of epilepsy that is not satisfactorily controlled by other antiepileptic drugs and it is the first-line treatment for West syndrome.

Irreversible constriction of the visual field (tunnel vision) and psychiatric adverse drug reactions make vigabatrin a drug of last choice in the treatment of epilepsy. Other adverse drug reactions are mainly CNS-related, such as drowsiness, dizziness, headache and ataxia.

Clinical case studies

> ### CASE STUDY 10.1

John is a 50-year-old man; he has been suffering from complex partial and generalised tonic-clonic seizures since a road traffic accident 30 years ago. Since then he has been prescribed phenytoin and has become free from generalised tonic-clonic seizures and only suffers infrequent complex partial seizures.

His seizures have been well controlled for the last 20 years with monotherapy of phenytoin 300 mg; however, he experienced a tonic-clonic seizure last week after a holiday in the USA. He was then admitted to hospital for further investigation. John weighs 70 kg and is 170 cm in height, with no other medical condition or other medication.

Would you request TDM? Why?
Yes; noncompliance during the holiday could be the cause of the seizure.

The SHO requests TDM and the pre-dose result is 7 mg/L; he wants to increase the dose of phenytoin and asks for your advice.

What would you recommend?
It is important to check the compliance when the patient was on holiday. If the 'low level' is caused by noncompliance, increasing the dose would not be appropriate.

Since John experienced status epilepticus owing to noncompliance when he was young, he has been taking his phenytoin regularly and he confirms that he was taking his phenytoin as usual while he was in the USA. The SHO therefore decides to increase the dose of phenytoin and asks you to calculate the dose in order to achieve a plasma level of 10 mg/mL (lower end of the usual therapeutic range).

We can use the population data and equation (10.2) to estimate the new dose (R_{new}): the population K_m is 5.7 mg/L in adults.

$$C_p^{ss} = K_m \frac{R \times F \times S}{V_m - (R \times F \times S)}$$

$$7 = 5.7 \times \frac{300 \times 1 \times 0.92}{V_m - (300 \times 1 \times 0.92)}$$

$$V_m = 500$$

$$10 = 5.7 \times \frac{Y \times 1 \times 0.92}{500 - (Y \times 1 \times 0.92)}$$

R_{new} = 345 mg; i.e. 350 mg tablets or capsules

However, it is important to remember that the population pharmacokinetic may not be right for John.

John is discharged with phenytoin 350 mg and a follow-up appointment is due a month later.

$\rightarrow$

CASE STUDY 10.1 (continued)

When John returns for his follow up appointment, he reports that he has had no tonic-clonic seizures, but he has had frequent complex partial seizures. The SHO takes another TDM and the result is 12 mg/mL. In order to help John to become seizure-free, the SHO considers increasing the phenytoin dose by another 50 mg, and asks for your advice.

For John's clinical situation, it is probably not necessary to calculate the dose, and the SHO could increase the dose by another 25 mg and observe the clinical response. However, a further 50 mg increment could be too much, so you could check the estimated concentration by obtaining V_m and K_m for John.

We can estimate John's K_m and V_m using equation (10.2). For 300 mg phenytoin, the plasma level was 7 mg/L. Applying equation (10.2):

$$7 = K_m \times \frac{300 \times 1 \times 0.92}{V_m - (300 \times 1 \times 0.92)}$$

$$V_m = (276K_m/7) + 276 \tag{10.3}$$

$$V_m = 39.4K_m + 276$$

For 350 mg phenytoin, the plasma level was 12 mg/L:

$$12 = K_m \times \frac{350 \times 1 \times 0.92}{V_m - (350 \times 1 \times 0.92)} \tag{10.4}$$

Combining equations (10.3) and (10.4):

$$12 = \frac{322K_m}{[(39.4K_m + 276) - 322]}$$

$$12 = \frac{322K_m}{[39.4K_m - 46]}$$

$$472.8K_m - 552 = 322K_m$$

$$K_m = 3.7$$

Substituting $K_m = 3.7$ into equation (10.3):

$$V_m = (39.4 \times 3.7) + 276$$

$$V_m = 422, \text{ round to } 420$$

If the dose were increased by 50 mg to 400 mg, we would expect to have the level:

$$C_p^{ss} = \frac{3.7[400 \times 1 \times 0.92]}{[420 - (400 \times 1 \times 0.92)]}$$

$$= 26 \text{ mg/L}$$

$\longrightarrow$

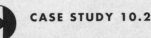

CASE STUDY 10.1 (continued)

In contrast, if we used the population data:

$$C_p^{ss} = \frac{5.7[400 \times 1 \times 0.92]}{[500 - (400 \times 1 \times 0.92)]}$$

$$= 16\,mg/L$$

A dosage of 400 mg daily is likely to cause a toxic effect, so it would be appropriate to try increasing the dose by 25 mg instead, and we can apply equation (10.2) to estimate the level:

$$C_p^{ss} = \frac{3.7[375 \times 1 \times 0.2]}{[420 - (375 \times 1 \times 0.92)]}$$

$$= 17\,mg/L$$

Since the dose was increased to 375 mg, John has become seizure-free.

CASE STUDY 10.2

Susan is a 70-year-old woman. She developed complex partial seizures after she suffered from a stroke 3 months ago; 4 weeks ago carbamazepine was initiated and increased to 200 mg three times a day, and she has not had a seizure since then. In her regular appointment with the hospital, she complains of dizziness and double vision in the morning, which wears off and then recurs after lunch.

Is there any indication for TDM?
Yes. Dizziness and double vision are dose-dependent reactions (Type A) to carbamazepine; therefore TDM would be useful.

The pre-dose plasma level is found to be 5 mg/L. As the plasma level is not particularly high and the seizures are under control, the doctor asks for your advice to deal with side-effects. What would you suggest?

Although 4–10 mg/L is the usual guide for using carbamazepine, some patients may experience adverse drug reactions at the lower end of the range; similarly, some patients may need higher concentrations to achieve the therapeutic effects. As Susan is likely to experience adverse drug reaction to carbamazepine, a small dose reduction may be required. However, Susan is taking carbamazepine three times a day and the adverse drug reactions seem

→

CASE STUDY 10.2 (continued)

to be related to the morning and afternoon doses. Type A reactions such as dizziness and diplopia are frequently associated with peak plasma level; switching to a twice-daily dose of a slow-release formulation might avoid the high peaks and reduce the likelihood of dose-dependent adverse drug reactions. However, the bioavailability of slow-release formulations is lower than that of regular-release formulations, so close monitoring is required and dose incrementation may be necessary.

Her doctor decides to change to 300 mg twice a day of a slow-release formulation; the subsequent plasma level is 4 mg/L and Susan experiences no more dizziness and diplopia, and the seizures are well-controlled.

CASE STUDY 10.3

Joseph is a 45-year-old man with epilepsy; he has had epilepsy since 7 years of age. His seizures have been controlled by phenytoin 350 mg daily, carbamazepine 300 mg three times a day and phenobarbital 30 mg at night. Recently, he has found himself very slow most of the time. You are his local hospital pharmacist and he has asked for your advice.

What is your advice?
Research has shown that about 60–70% patients with epilepsy can be treated adequately by monotherapy; only patients with severe epilepsy require polypharmacy. You could advise him to see his consultant and consider monotherapy.

His consultant agrees with your suggestion and starts a phenobarbital withdrawal programme. Why did the consultant choose the phenobarbital?
Firstly, phenobarbital probably has more nonspecific CNS-suppression effects than the other two medications. Secondly, 30 mg is a very low dose for epilepsy treatment, so it is probably not necessary at all.

Would you recommend TDM for Joseph?
Yes. Removal of phenobarbital would reduce the metabolism of the other two drugs, so it is necessary to monitor the plasma levels and adjust dosages accordingly.

→

CASE STUDY 10.3 (continued)

Four months later, Joseph returns and has successfully stopped phenobarbital. The consultant decides to initiate a programme to obtain monotherapy for Joseph. Which drug would you recommend?
Phenytoin would probably be the one to withdraw. On the basis of the current evidence, carbamazepine and phenytoin have similar efficacy, but the non-linear pharmacokinetics of phenytoin make it a difficult medication to use. Furthermore, the safety profile of carbamazepine is more favourable.

The consultant decides to withdraw phenytoin gradually and continues to monitor the plasma level of carbamazepine. A few months later, Joseph is on carbamazepine monotherapy and feels more alert.

CASE STUDY 10.4

Jennifer is a 40-year-old woman; she has had epilepsy since she was 10. She has been on carbamazepine 400 mg three times a day. A month ago, she was prescribed lamotrigine to control her seizure and since the last lamotrigine dose increment to 100 mg twice daily she has started to experience dizziness, double vision and unsteadiness. The TDM results show no change in carbamazepine plasma level before and after lamotrigine was started.

What are the likely reasons for the dizziness, double vision and unsteadiness?
The cause is probably an interaction between lamotrigine and carbamazepine. Some literature reports suggest that the level of active carbamazepine metabolite is increased, causing adverse drug reactions; however, these findings were not confirmed by subsequent studies. Most people believe it is a pharmacodynamic interaction.

How would you deal with these adverse drug reactions?
As these reactions are dose-dependent (Type A reactions), a slight dose reduction of carbamazepine can stop them.

References/Further reading

French J A, Kanner A M, Bautista J *et al.* (2004a). Efficacy and tolerability of the new antiepileptic drugs II: treatment of refractory epilepsy: Report of the Therapeutics and Technology Assessment Subcommittee and Quality Standards Subcommittee of the American Academy of Neurology and the American Epilepsy Society. *Neurology* 62(8): 1261–1273.

French J A, Kanner A M, Bautista J *et al.* (2004b). Efficacy and tolerability of the new antiepileptic drugs I: treatment of new onset epilepsy: Report of the Therapeutics and Technology Assessment Subcommittee and Quality Standards Subcommittee of the American Academy of Neurology and the American Epilepsy Society. *Neurology* 62(8): 1252–1260.

Johannessen S I, Battino D, Berry D J *et al.* (2003). Therapeutic drug monitoring of the newer antiepileptic drugs. *Ther Drug Monit* 25(3): 347–363.

NICE (2004). *Clinical Guideline 20. The epilepsies: the diagnosis and management of the epilepsies in adults and children in primary and secondary care.* http://www.nice.org.uk/page.aspx?0=227586 (accessed 16/11/2005).

Patsalos P N, Perucca E (2003). Clinically important drug interactions in epilepsy: general features and interactions between antiepileptic drugs. *Lancet Neurol* 2(6): 347–356.

Walker R, Edward R (2002). *Clinical Pharmacy and Therapeutics*, 3rd edn. London: Churchill Livingstone.

11

Ciclosporin

Douglas Maclean

Aims and learning outcomes

The aims of this chapter are:

- To outline briefly the mechanism of action of ciclosporin.
- To examine factors that cause intra- and inter-patient variability with ciclosporin.
- To detail various approaches to therapeutic drug monitoring.

Introduction

Ciclosporin is a powerful, steroid-sparing immunosuppressant agent originally isolated from the fungus *Tolpocladium inflatum* Gams (Borel *et al.*, 1976). Its use in human medicine has grown extensively since its clinical introduction in the late 1970s. Over the past twenty years, ciclosporin has become the cornerstone of immunosuppression in transplantation of bone marrow, heart, liver, kidney and other organs. In renal transplantation it has been used as a monotherapy or in combination with other agents to prevent rejection of the transplanted organ and it has increasing applications in the management of autoimmune diseases.

How ciclosporin works

To enable activation, T-lymphocytes require two signals, the first delivered through the clonally expressed T-cell receptor (TCR) and the second mediated by co-stimulatory interactions between the B7 and CD40 groups of molecules on the antigen-presenting cell and between the CD28 and CD40 ligands on the T-cell (Jenkins and Schwarz, 1987; Schwarz, 1992). These two signals are essential for the phosphorylation of a number of cytoplasmic proteins, resulting in a sustained rise in intracellular calcium (Cantrell, 1996).

A cascade of reactions is triggered, resulting in the immunological activation of T-lymphocytes in conjunction with production of certain

Table 11.1 Pharmacokinetic parameters for ciclosporin

Parameter	Value
Bioavailability (%)	8–60
First-pass metabolism (%)	10–27
Enterohepatic recirculation	Metabolites only
Hepatic metabolism (%)	99
Clearance (L/h/kg)	0.15–0.7
V_d^{ss} (L/kg)^a	0.1–1.7
$t_{1/2\alpha}$ (h)^b	2.9–15.8
$t_{1/2\beta}$ (h)^c	2.9
Biliary excretion (%)	>90

^{a} V_d^{ss} = volume of distribution at steady state.
^{b} $t_{1/2\alpha}$ = absorption phase half life.
^{c} $t_{1/2\beta}$ = elimination half life.

growth factors, which drive the cell into the growth cycle. Foremost among the growth factors is the pro-inflammatory cytokine interleukin-2 (IL-2). The key effects of ciclosporin are to impair production of IL-2 and retard lymphocytic proliferation.

A potent calcineurin inhibitor, ciclosporin exhibits a narrow therapeutic range with complex pharmacokinetics. Pharmacokinetic parameters for ciclosporin in healthy human adult volunteers exhibit large ranges, as shown in Table 11.1. Marked intrapatient (up to twofold) and interpatient (greater than threefold) variability in area-under-the-curve (AUC) estimations is found even under standardised conditions (Scott and Higenbottam, 1988).

Ciclosporin for oral administration was originally formulated in an oily solution that contained excipients including corn oil, polyethoxylated castor oil and ethanol, available as Sandimmun. Oral absorption from the Sandimmun formulation was extremely erratic. The unpredictable pharmacokinetic behaviour of ciclosporin resulted in poor correlations between trough level concentrations (TLC) and the AUC with Sandimmun. This led to practical difficulties in dosing patients. The re-formulated microemulsion Neoral developed in the mid-1990s exhibits closer correlation between TLC and AUC. Because of this association, it is believed, optimal immunosuppression may be achieved with minimal adverse effects.

Absorption

Ciclosporin is slowly and incompletely absorbed from the gastrointestinal tract. Absorption occurs predominantly in the small intestine (Drew *et al.*, 1992).

Renal transplant recipients with an oral bioavailability <25% had lower renal transplant survival at one year. These patients were less likely to have a rejection-free year compared with patients absorbing a larger proportion of the dose. Following oral administration, ciclosporin absorption is highly variable and can be retarded by a variety of factors including presystemic metabolism caused by cytochrome oxidase enzymes located in the enteral mucosa, the presence of food in the gastrointestinal tract, concurrent medications and biliary flow.

The influence of P-glycoprotein-mediated transport of ciclosporin from the enterocytes back into the gut lumen is of major importance (Bistrup *et al.*, 2001). Notable ethnic differences in absorption of ciclosporin have been reported in various population groups including Afro-Caribbeans (Stein *et al.*, 2001) and Asians (Chowbay *et al.*, 2003), who express higher levels of P-glycoprotein (Pollak *et al.*, 1999; Min *et al.*, 2000).

Absorption of ciclosporin can be reduced in diabetic gastroparesis, grossly impaired in cystic fibrosis (Cooney *et al.*, 1990), and altered markedly, especially by drugs affecting gastrointestinal motility such as metoclopramide (Wadwha *et al.*, 1987).

Following oral administration, ciclosporin appears in the blood after 0–0.9 h. The reported absorption half-life ranges from 0.5 to 2 h (Lindberg, 1986), confirmed in further studies (Grevel, 1986).

Ciclosporin blood concentrations measured 2 h following oral administration are allegedly more highly correlated with the AUC than are whole-blood trough levels.

Distribution

Significant sequestration of ciclosporin occurs in erythrocytes – around 60%. With chronic dosing there appears to be low passage across the blood–brain barrier. A large fraction of ciclosporin that crosses the blood–brain barrier is concentrated in the cerebral microvasculature. Ciclosporin neurotoxicity despite therapeutic blood levels has been reported; this was reversible on withdrawal of the drug (Hughes, 1990).

Metabolism

It may be anticipated that ciclosporin, as a peptide, would be metabolised extensively in the gastrointestinal tract both enzymatically and by intestinal flora. Being N-methylated, seven of ciclosporin's amino acids protect the cyclic peptide from intestinal degradation (Loor *et al.*, 2002). Ciclosporin is metabolised predominantly hepatically, by the cytochrome P450 111a4 enzyme system, to a large number of metabolites, some of which are active.

Elimination

Clearance of ciclosporin from the body is predominantly hepatic, via the hepatobiliary tract. Ciclosporin is a drug with a low to intermediate extraction ratio. It does not undergo excessive first-pass metabolism and extraction of the drug varies from 17% to 50% of the dose (Kahan, 1985).

Monitoring of ciclosporin in transplant patients

An extremely comprehensive review of the methods employed for the therapeutic monitoring of ciclosporin in transplant recipients is cited by Dumont and Ensom (2000).

Trough concentration monitoring

Monitoring of the trough level concentration (TLC) of ciclosporin in whole blood (TCM) remains by far the most convenient, practical, simple and routine method of monitoring ciclosporin in transplant recipients. At the Lake Louise Consensus Conference on Ciclosporin Monitoring in Organ Transplantation, the consensus panel detailed several analytical techniques and numerous therapeutic ranges for differing types of analyses of ciclosporin in whole blood (Oellerrich *et al.*, 1995). Ciclosporin whole-blood level data presented at the Lake Louise Conference were based on patients who had been administered Sandimmun.

Neoral was not commercially available in the UK until the mid-1990s. Ciclosporin TLC remains the most universally accepted index of ciclosporin measured in blood but it fails to reflect accurately the exposure of the body to the drug (Kasiske *et al.*, 1988). Single ciclosporin whole-blood trough levels correlate poorly with AUC.

Despite the commercial availability of Sandimmun since the early 1980s, or more recently of Neoral since the mid-1990s, a fixed therapeutic range for ciclosporin in any area of organ transplantation remains ill defined. The literature states that ciclosporin is a drug with a narrow therapeutic range, but controversy arises from the loose correlations between TLC, therapeutic range, acute toxicity and efficacy.

The complexities of immunosuppressive strategies and concomitant medications, many of which can interact with ciclosporin, undoubtedly further complicate identification of a well-defined therapeutic range for ciclosporin. Given the widespread use of ciclosporin in organ transplantation over the last two decades it is unfortunate that, to date, no large-scale global multicentre studies have clarified the therapeutic range(s) for whole-blood trough concentrations of the drug in varying types of organ transplantation.

With respect to TCM, the pursuit of perfection in analytical techniques is somewhat pointless if the parameter measured correlates neither with pharmacological efficacy nor with clinical outcome.

Regardless of what technique is used, ciclosporin dose adjustment must ultimately be made according to a patient's response and not to a laboratory level.

AUC monitoring

Monitoring of the area under the concentration–time curve (AUC) provides a more accurate indication of exposure of the body to the drug. AUC monitoring is logistically more complex, involving the administration of a dose of a drug followed by serial blood sampling. Measured whole-blood concentrations can then used to determine the AUC, usually using the trapezoidal rule.

Attempts were made at estimation of pretransplantation ciclosporin pharmacokinetic parameters in a series of 36 renal transplant recipients. Characterisation of pretransplantation pharmacokinetic parameters was then performed to forecast optimal posttransplantation ciclosporin dosing. The study was designed to demonstrate that AUC monitoring was superior to TCM (Grevel *et al.*, 1989). Correlation analysis was based on 71 paired observations of ciclosporin measured by polyclonal radioimmunoassay in 36 patients for 36 months. AUC, but not TLC, was correlated significantly with the administered oral dose. The caveat of this principle is that AUC monitoring must outperform TLC monitoring as long as the principles of linear pharmacokinetics are not violated. A subsequent study in renal transplantation patients showed that interpatient variability could be counterbalanced by dosage individualisation through the use of AUC monitoring (Grevel and Kahan, 1991).

Using high-pressure liquid chromatography (HPLC) analyses of blood in 45 patients, Kasiske *et al.* (1988) studied AUCs at 1, 4 and 12 weeks after renal transplantation. Eleven AUC evaluations were performed less than 2 weeks prior to acute rejection episodes. The pre-rejection concentration profiles showed significantly lower maximum concentrations ($p < 0.01$) and 21% lower dose-adjusted AUCs than did the other concentration–time profiles ($p < 0.05$). However, although the 24-h trough concentrations were 20% lower in rejecting patients, this difference did not achieve statistical significance (Lindholm *et al.*, 1995). A further study of 1868 pharmacokinetic profiles was performed during the first 90 posttransplantation days of 160 renal transplant recipients. There was an increased rate of acute rejection episodes among patients displaying initially low steady-state whole-blood concentrations of ciclosporin during intravenous infusion ($C^{ss} < 350$ ng/mL; $C_{av} < 400$ ng/mL) and/or high values of whole-blood clearance rates ($CL > 325$ mL/min) (Kahan et al., 1995).

AUC can be useful to characterise abnormal or atypical absorption patterns, e.g. diabetic gastroparesis or cystic fibrosis, and can be useful as a predictor of clinical outcomes (Grevel and Kahan, 1991), in addition to allowing characterisation of pharmacokinetic parameters. The consensus is that AUC is superior to TCM, although this remains to be confirmed by prospective studies demonstrating clear advantages in terms of outcome data.

AUC monitoring is labour-intensive, costly, inconvenient for patients and not practical in the context of a busy outpatient clinic.

Limited sampling strategies

An alternative technique to AUC monitoring is 'limited sampling strategies' (LSSs). These have been developed as they allow the determination of pharmacokinetic parameters.

Limited sampling strategy has been developed from full AUC calculations in sample populations. Stepwise multiple regression analysis is then performed on the concentration–time points. The points that do not correlate well with AUC are removed until a regression equation consisting of few concentration–time points remains. The equation must have a high coefficient of determination associated with it. Mathematical bias and precision should also be calculated in order to assess the predictive performance of the limited sampling strategy. A number of limited sampling strategy equations have been derived for a variety of transplant patients taking Neoral (see Table 11.2).

Limited sampling strategies offer a clinically useful alternative to full AUC determinations. No studies are currently available supporting the superiority of the technique over whole-blood trough concentration monitoring. Validation of a LSS study in a given centre should be performed using the techniques proposed by Sheiner and Beal (1981).

Ciclosporin absorption profiling

The use of a single ciclosporin blood concentration data point 2 h after administration of an oral dose of Neoral (C_2) has recently provoked

Table 11.2 Summary of selected limited sampling strategies for monitoring ciclosporin

Reference	Patient group	AUC interval[a] (h)	Equation[b]
Amante and Kahan (1996)	Renal adult	12	$AUC = 2.4C_2 + 7.7C_6 + 195.8$
Cooney et al. (1996)	Liver paediatric	8	$AUC = 10.19C_0 + 4.47C_3 + 749.7$
Foradori et al. (1995)	Renal adult	12	$AUC = 0.681C_1 + 1.859C_{2.5} + 3.411C_5 + 791.74$
Gaspari et al. (1997)	Renal adult	12	$AUC = 5.189C_0 + 1.267C_1 + 4.15C_3 + 135.079$
Johnston et al. (1996)	Renal adult	12	$AUC = 1.96C_2 + 11.5C_8 + 355.2$
Keown et al. (1996)	Renal adult	12	$AUC = 1.84C_0 + 4.39C_2 + 312.66$
Lemire et al. (1998)	Renal adult	12	$AUC = 1.023C_1 + 13.10C_6 + 242$
Marsh (1999)	Renal adult	12	$AUC = 6(C_0 + C_4)$
Meier-Kresche et al. (1998)	Renal adult/ paediatric	8	$AUC = 1.84C_2 + 4.39C_4 + 129$
Primmett et al. (1998)	Renal adult	12	$AUC = 12.34C_0 + 2.48C_2 + 441.42$
Serafinowicz et al. (1996)	Renal adult	12	$AUC = 9.131C_0 + 0.784C_1 + 2.617C_2 + 193.561$

[a] AUC = area under the concentration–time curve ($h\ ng\ mL^{-1}$).
[b] C_n = whole-blood concentration at n hours.

considerable interest among pharmacokineticists and physicians. The rationale is that a ciclosporin concentration measured 2 h following an oral dose of ciclosporin is more highly correlated with the AUC in the first 4 h following oral dosing than is a TLC measurement.

In a study of 30 stable heart transplant recipients it was demonstrated that C_2 correlated better than TLC with the AUC_{0-4h} ($r = 0.91$ vs 0.63), when C_2 levels remained in the range 300–600 ng/mL. During 6-month follow-up of these patients, the C_2 group were noted to require lower Neoral doses, had a reduction in serum creatinine levels, and lacked evidence of endomyocardial biopsy-proven acute rejection (Cantarovich et al., 1998).

A further study in 35 stable adult liver transplant recipients supported the superiority of C_2 versus TLC monitoring, confirming the

Table 11.3 C_2 monitoring targets in liver and renal transplantation

Months post transplantation	Proposed C_2 targets (ng/mL) based on currently available data
	Adult liver transplantation
0–6	1000
6–12	800
>12	600
	Adult renal transplantation
0–1	1700
1–2	1500
2–3	1300
3–6	1100
6–12	800
12+	600

close association of C_2 with AUC_{0-4h} ($r = 0.92$ vs $r = 0.40$), also showing that C_2 levels in the range of 300–600 ng/mL resulted in lower Neoral doses and greater clinical benefit, defined as the absence of rejection with no increase in serum creatinine at 7-month follow-up (Cantarovich et al., 1998). In a multicentre study INT-06 (Levy et al., 2002), 307 de novo liver transplant recipients were randomised to C_2 ($n = 158$) or C_0 ($n = 148$) monitoring strategies. Dose adjustment of Neoral was made to predefined ranges: $C_2 = 850$–1400 ng/mL, $C_0 = 250$–400 ng/mL. Overall incidence of acute rejection was lower for the C_2 group (26.5%) than for the C_0 group (33.5%), but the difference did not reach statistical significance. The proportion of biopsy-proven rejection episodes at 12 months was noted to be 47% (C_2 group) vs 70% (C_0 group) ($p = 0.02$). The authors conclude that Neoral monitoring in de novo liver transplantation reduces the incidence and severity of acute rejection compared with C_2 monitoring (see Table 11.3).

For optimal outcome, C_2 target levels should be achieved by day 5 post transplantation. If the C_2 target level is less than the desired target level on day 5, a C_2 and a C_6 sample should be assayed to assess for delayed absorption. If the C_6 level is less than the C_2 level.

Accuracy of C_2 blood sampling

There is a 15-minute 'window of opportunity' before and after the 2 h time point during which the C_2 sample can be taken in order to remain within a 10% margin of error (Saint-Marcoux et al., 2003). Anecdotally, the total daily dosage should not exceed 15 mg per kg body weight per day unless abnormally low absorption of ciclosporin has been demonstrated, e.g. C_6 level $<$ C_2 level. Beyond this 15-minute window, the level of error is considered too high for a meaningful adjustment to Neoral dosing. In most instances, C_2 targets do not require adjustment for different immunoassay types currently available.

The Neoral C_2 dose adjustment formula is as follows:

$$\text{New Neoral dose} = \text{Old Neoral dose} \times \frac{\text{Target } C_2 \text{ level}}{\text{Current } C_2 \text{ level}}$$

Neoral dosage adjustments based on C_2 levels must only be made if the C_2 measurement is taken within the 15-minute 'window of opportunity' described above.

Although the results of the MO2ART study are awaited, further prospective randomised controlled studies comparing ciclosporin whole-blood trough concentrations with ciclosporin 2 h concentrations are required to evaluate the long-term efficacy in reduction of acute organ rejection and reduction in the adverse effects of chronic ciclosporin therapy.

Other recent studies with Neoral (Kovarik *et al.*, 1994; Kahan *et al.*, 1995) have confirmed the earlier work of Cantarovich, provoking further interest in C_2 as a more informative surrogate index of body exposure to this drug.

Acknowledgement

Special thanks to Graeme Smith for his helpful comments.

References/Further reading

Amante J, Kahan B D (1996). Abbreviated area-under-the-curve strategy for monitoring cyclosporine microemulsion therapy in immediate posttransplant period. *Clin Chem* 42: 1294–1296.

Beveridge T, Gratwohl A, Michot F *et al.* (1981). Cyclosporin A: pharmacokinetics after a single dose in man and serum levels after multiple dosing in recipients of allogeneic bone marrow grafts.*Curr Ther Res* 30: 5–18.

Bistrup C, Finn T N, Unni E J, Dieperink H (2001). Effect of grapefruit juice on Sandimmun Neoral® absorption among stable renal allograft recipients. *Nephrol Dial Transplant* 16: 373–377.

Borel J F, Feurer C, Gubler H C, Stahelin H (1976). Biological effects of cyclosporine A: a new lymphocytic agent. *Agents Actions* 6: 468–475.

Cantarovich M, Besner J G, Barkun J S *et al.* (1998). Two hour cyclosporine level determination is the appropriate tool to monitor Neoral® therapy. *Clin Transplant* 12: 243–249.

Cantrell D F (1996). T-cell antigen receptor signal transduction pathways. *Annu Rev Immunol* 15: 707–747.

Chowbay B, Cumaraswamy S, Cheung Y B, Zhou Q, Lee E J (2003). Genetic polymorphisms in MDR1 and CYP3A4 genes in Asians and the influence of MDR1 haplotypes on cyclosporine disposition in heart transplant recipients. *Pharmacogenetics* 13(2): 89–95.

Cooney G F, Fiel S B, Shaw L M *et al.* (1990). Bioavailability of oral cyclosporine A in heart-lung transplant candidates with cystic fibrosis. *Transplantation* 49: 821–3.

Cooney G F, Lum B L, Meligeni, J A *et al.* (1996). Pharmacokinetics of a microemulsion formulation of cyclosporine in paediatric liver transplant patients. *Transplant Proc* 28: 2270–2272.

Drew J, Beglinger C, Kissel T. (1992). The absorption of cyclosporine in the human gastrointestinal tract. *Br J Clin Pharmacol* 33: 39–43.

Dumont R J, Ensom M (2000). Methods for clinical monitoring of cyclosporin in transplant patients. *Clin Pharmacokinet* 38(5): 427–447.

Foradori A C, Martinez L, Elberg A *et al.* (1995). Preliminary pharmacokinetic evaluation of a new galenical formulation of oral cyclosporine A: Neoral®. *Transplant Proc* 27: 1813–1814.

Gaspari F, Anedda M F, Signorini O *et al.* (1997). Prediction of cyclosporine area under the curve using a three point sampling strategy after Neoral administration. *J Am Soc Nephrol* 8: 647–652.

Grevel J (1986). Absorption of cyclosporine A after oral dosing. *Transplantation Proc* 18 (Suppl 5): 9–15.

Grevel J, Kahan B D (1991). Area under the curve monitoring of cyclosporine therapy: the early post-transplant period. *Ther Drug Monit* 13: 89–95.

Grevel J, Welsh M S, Kahan B D (1989). Cyclosporin monitoring in renal transplantation: under the curve monitoring is superior to trough level monitoring. *Ther Drug Monit* 11: 246–248.

Hughes R L (1990). Cyclosporine-related central nervous system toxicity in cardiac transplantation. *N Engl J Med* 323: 420–421.

Jenkins M K, Scharz R H (1987). Antigen presentation by chemically modified splenocytes induces antigen-specific T cell unresponsiveness *in vitro* and *in vivo*. *J Exp Med* 165: 302–319.

Johnston A, Kovarik J M, Mueller E A *et al.* (1996). Predicting patients' exposure to cyclosporine. *Transplant Int* 9: S305–S307.

Kahan B D (1985). Individualisation of cyclosporine therapy using pharmacokinetic and pharmacodynamic parameters *Transplantation* 41: 459–464.

Kahan B D, Welsh M, Rutzky L (1995). Challenges in cyclosporine therapy: the role of therapeutic monitoring by area under the curve monitoring. *Ther Drug Monit* 17: 621–624.

Kasiske B L, Heim-Duthoy K, Rao K V *et al.* (1988). The relationship between cyclosporine pharmacokinetic parameters and subsequent acute rejection in renal transplant recipients.*Transplantation* 46: 716–722.

Keown P, Landsberg D, Halloran P et al. (1996). A randomised prospective multi-centre pharmacoepidemiologic study of cyclosporine microemulsion in stable renal graft recipients. *Transplantation* 42: 1744–1752.

Kovarik J M, Mueller E A, van Bree et al. (1994). Reduced inter and intraindividual variability in cyclosporine pharmacokinetics from a microemulsion formulation. *J Pharm Sci* 83: 444–446.

Lemire J, Capparelli D, MacDonald D et al. (1998). Estimated area-under-the curve monitoring of Neoral in a stable paediatric renal transplant population: one year experience. *Transplant Proc* 30: 1983–1984.

Levy G, Thervet E, Lake J, Uchida K (2002). Patient management by Neoral C2 monitoring: an international consensus. *Transplantation* 73(9, suppl.): 512–518.

Lindberg A, Odlind B, Tufveson G, Lindstrom B, Gabrielson J (1986). The pharmacokinetics of cyclosporine A in uraemic patients. *Transplantation Proc* 18 (Suppl 5): 144–152.

Lindholm A, Sawe J (1995). Pharmacokinetics and therapeutic drug monitoring of immunosuppressants. *Ther Drug Monit* 17: 570–573.

Lindholm A, Henricsson S, Lind M, Dahlqvist R (1988). Intraindividual variability in the relative systemic availability of cyclosporine after oral dosing. *Eur J Clin Pharmacol* 34: 461–464.

Loor F, Tiberhien F, Wenandy T, Didier A, Traber R (2002). Cyclosporins: structure–activity relationships for the inhibition of the human MDR1 P-glycoprotein ABC transporter. *J Med Chem* 45(21): 4598–4612.

Marsh C L (1999). Abbreviated pharmacokinetic profiles in area under the curve monitoring of cyclosporine therapy in de novo renal with Sandimmune or Neoral. *Ther Drug Monit* 21: 27–34.

Meier-Kriesche H U, Kaplan B, Brannan P et al. (1998). A limited sampling strategy for the estimation of eight-hour Neoral areas under the curve in renal transplantation. *Ther Drug Monit* 20: 401–407.

Min D I, Lee M, Ku Y M, Flannigan M (2000). Gender-dependent racial differences in disposition of cyclosporine among healthy African–American and white volunteers. *Clin Pharmacol Ther* 68(5): 478–486.

Oellerich M, Armstrong V W, Kahan B et al. (1995). Lake Louise Consensus Conference on Cyclosporin Monitoring in Organ Transplantation: Report of the Consensus Panel. *Ther Drug Monit* 16: 642–654.

Pollak R, Wong R L, Chang R T (1999). Cyclosporine bioavailability of Neoral® and Sandimmune® in white and black *de novo* renal transplant recipients. Neoral Study Group. *Ther Drug Monit* 21(6); 661–663.

Primmett D R N, Levine M, Kovarik J M et al. (1998). Cyclosporine monitoring in patients with renal transplants: two or three-point methods that estimate area under the curve are superior to trough levels in predicting drug exposure. *Ther Drug Monit* 20: 276–283.

Saint-Marcoux F, Rousseau A, Le Meur Y et al. (2003). Influence of sampling-time error on cyclosporine measurements nominally at 2 hours after administration orally. *Clin Chem* 58(12): 813–820.

Schwarz R H (1992). Co-stimulation of T lymphocytes: the role of CD28,CTL A-4 and B7/BB1 in interleukin-2 production in immunotherapy. *Cell* 71: 1065–1068.

Scott J P, Higenbottam T W (1988). Adverse reactions and interactions of cyclosporin. *Med Toxicol* 3: 107–127.

Serafinowicz A, Gaciong Z, Baczkowska T *et al.* (1996). Limited sampling strategy to estimate exposure to cyclosporine A in renal allograft recipients treated with Sandimmun-Neoral. *Transplant Proc* 28: 3138–3139.

Sheiner L B, Beal S L (1981). Some suggestions for measuring predictive performance. *J Pharmacokinet Biopharm* 45: 389–394.

Stein C M, Sadeque A J, Murray J J, Wandel C, Kim R B, Wood A J (2001). Cyclosporin pharmacokinetics and pharmacodynamics in African American and white subjects. *Clin Pharmacol Ther* 69(5): 317–323.

Wadwha N K, Schroeder T J, O'Flaherty *et al.* (1987). The effect of oral metoclopramide on the absorption of cyclosporine. *Transplantation* 43: 211–213.

12

Clinical case studies

Andrzej Kostrzewski

Aims and learning outcomes

This chapter includes six actual case studies of patients who demonstrate particular clinical therapeutic drug monitoring (TDM) problems with five drugs that are routinely monitored and that have been discussed in the previous chapters.

The purposes of the cases are:

- To allow the reader to use the cases as self-assessment exercises in the use of pharmacokinetic calculations.
- To illustrate how pharmacokinetics can be used to make professional judgements in health care.
- To provide a set of tools for the education of others.

Each case study is based on real patients who have been prescribed the drugs listed in Table 12.1. The case studies are of two formats, either a report using a time line of a problem or a question/answer format.

Table 12.1 Summary of case studies

Case	Drug	Report format	Problem illustrated
1	Digoxin	Time line	Interpretation of toxic measured levels compared to population prediction
2	Aminophylline	Time line	Infusion dose recommendation and infusion to oral switch
3	Gentamicin	Question/answer	TDM in liver disease and problems in sampling
4	Phenytoin	Question/answer	Population prediction and toxicity due to protein binding changes
5	Phenytoin/ carbamazepine	Time line	Prediction of levels and effect of pregnancy
6	Digoxin	Time line	Drug toxicity and reasons for decreased toxicity

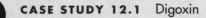

CASE STUDY 12.1 Digoxin

A 78-year-old woman weighing 47 kg was complaining of sickness and was vomiting. The GP requested a serum digoxin level because her pulse was 50 bpm. A differential diagnosis of digoxin toxicity and gastritis was made. The dose of digoxin was 0.25 mg daily. The patient was also taking co-amilozide, one in the morning, and metoprolol 50 mg twice daily. The serum creatinine and potassium were measured and the results were:

Serum potassium   4.1 mmol/L (normal range 3.5–5.2 mmol/L)
Serum creatinine   154 μmol/L (normal range 45–120 μmol/L)

A calculation of the digoxin concentration from standard formulae revealed that the concentration would be high.
Calculation of creatinine clearance:

$$\text{Creatinine clearance} = \frac{1.04 \times (140 - \text{Age}) \times \text{IBW}}{\text{Serum creatinne}}$$
$$= 19 \text{ mL/min}$$

The *digoxin clearance* was calculated from the formula generated by Kelman *et al.* (1982).

$$\text{Digoxin clearance} = (0.06 \times 19) + (0.02 \times 47)$$
$$= 2.5 \text{ L/h}$$

Therefore the predicted steady-state digoxin concentration was 3.2 ng/mL.
Laboratory result: Serum digoxin = 4.3 ng/mL
   When the digoxin sample was measured by the laboratory using RIA, the concentration was 4.3 ng/mL. The difference in the results may be due to assay inaccuracies at high concentrations, or to wrong assumptions in the assessment of the population parameters, or to other factors. The half-life was calculated to be 95 h, i.e. about 4 days. The doctor was phoned, with a recommendation to stop the drug. The drug was stopped and over the next 4 days the patient went into atrial fibrillation (AF), developed some ventricular ectopics and had a transient ischaemic attack (TIA).
   She was admitted to hospital, and a further serum digoxin was urgently requested by the casualty officer to ascertain the patient's status. However, because the pharmacokinetic parameters of this patient were available, the digoxin concentration on admission could be estimated.
   The estimated concentration was between 1.6 and 2.1 ng/mL, that is 50% of the previous concentration (one half-life or 4 days). The potassium concentration

$\rightarrow$

CASE STUDY 12.1 (continued)

was within the normal range and the serum creatinine had improved slightly to 120 μmol/L. This would indicate that the patient was unlikely to be digoxin toxic, but nevertheless fully digitalised. After consultation with the requesting doctor, it was decided that there was no need for the assay to be done urgently, and the patient could be restarted on digoxin at a maintenance dose of 125 μg daily.

A sample was taken for a retrospective measurement. The concentration was determined to be 1.2 ng/mL, indicating that the calculation was probably the more accurate estimate of the original concentration. The patient made a good recovery. The steady-state concentration of digoxin at this dose was calculated to be 1.3 ng/mL and, in fact, a sample taken 7 days later revealed a serum concentration of 1.4 ng/mL.

CASE STUDY 12.2 Aminophylline

Mr C.K., 37 years old, was admitted to hospital having suffered an exacerbation of his asthma. Following his admission he was started on an infusion of aminophylline 250 mg over 6 h, and after 48 h a serum level was measured. Mr C.K. is 175 cm (5 ft 9 in.) in height, weighs 79 kg, and is a nonsmoker.

Drug data, Phyllocontin Continus:	$k_a = 0.35 h^{-1}$
	$S = 0.79$
	$F = 1$
Assay result:	*Serum level = 6.7 μg/mL*
Target range:	*10–20 μg/mL*

Calculate population pharmacokinetic parameters

IBW = 50 + (2.3 ×every inch > 5 ft) = 50 + (2.3 × 9) = 71 kg

Use ABW since obesity <15%:

$$V_d = 0.5 \text{ L/kg actual body weight} = 39.5 \text{ L}$$
$$\text{Clearance (CL)} = 0.04 \text{ L/h/kg} \times \text{disease factor} = 0.04 \times 79$$
$$CL = 3.16 \text{ L/h}$$
$$k = CL/V_d = 0.08 \text{ h}^{-1}$$

$\rightarrow$

> **CASE STUDY12.2** (continued)

Assessment of patient parameters from the serum level data
Use population V_d:

$$V_d = 0.5 \times 79 = 39.5 \text{ L}$$

$$\text{Clearance} = \frac{\text{Dose} \times S \times F}{C_p^{ss} \times \tau} = \frac{250 \times 0.79 \times 1}{6.7 \times 6}$$

$$CL = 4.9 \text{ L/h}$$
$$k = 4.9/39.5 = 0.12 \text{ h}^{-1}$$

Interpretation
Comparison of the population data with Mr C.K.'s parameters indicates that this patient has a clearance that is considerably higher than expected, especially in view of the fact that he is a nonsmoker (smoking induces microsomal liver enzymes and therefore metabolism and clearance are increased).

Dosage recommendation
New maintenance dose

$$\text{New maintenance dose} = \frac{CL \times C_p^{ss} \times \tau}{S \times F}$$

$$\frac{500}{6} = \frac{4.9 \times C_p^{ss}}{0.79}$$
$$C_p^{ss} = 13.4 \text{ } \mu g/mL$$

A dose of 500 mg IV given over 6 h was therefore recommended and the doctor was advised to reassay 24 h later to confirm efficacy, which he did. The level was then found to be 11.8 μg/mL, which was prior to steady state and was therefore going to rise further. The doctor at this stage wished to start the patient on oral therapy and asked for a dosage recommendation.

Predicted plasma level
Assume the infusion was increased from 250 mg to 500 mg over 6 h, 16 h ago.

$$C_{pt} = C_p^0 \exp(-kt)$$
$$C_{pt} = 6.7 \text{ } e^{-0.12 \times 16} = 1 \text{ } \mu g/mL$$

$\rightarrow$

● **CASE STUDY 12.2** (continued)

C_p from new maintenance dose:

$$C_{pt} = \frac{D \times S \times F}{\tau \times CL} \times [1 - \exp(-kt)] \ \mu g/mL$$

$$= \frac{500 \times 0.79 \times 1}{6 \times 4.9} \times [1 - e^{-0.12 \times 16}] \ \mu g/mL$$

$$C_{pt} = 11.4 \ \mu g/mL$$

C_{pt} at time of sampling:

$$C_{pt} = 1 \ \mu g/mL + 11.4 \ \mu g/mL = 12.4 \ \mu g/mL$$

Predicted and observed levels are similar, indicating that the patient's parameters have not significantly altered.

Oral dose recommendation
An oral dose of 675 mg Phyllocontin Continus b.d. was advised.

$$\text{Time to peak} = \frac{1}{k_a - k} \ \ln\left\{\frac{k_a[1 - \exp(-k\tau)]}{k[1 - \exp(-k_a\tau)]}\right\}$$

$$= \frac{1}{0.35 - 0.12} \ \ln\left\{\frac{0.35[1 - e^{-0.12 \times 12}]}{0.12[1 - e^{-0.35 \times 12}]}\right\}$$

$$= 3.5 \ h$$

Predicted maximum concentration:

$$C_{p\,max}^{ss} = \frac{C_p^0 k_a}{k_a - k} \left\{\frac{\exp(-kt_{max}^{ss})}{1 - \exp(-k\tau)} - \frac{\exp(-k_a t_{max}^{ss})}{1 - \exp(-k_a\tau)}\right\}$$

$$C_p^0 = \frac{D \times S \times F}{V_d} = \frac{0.79 \times 1 \times 675}{39.5}$$

$$C_p^0 = 13.5 \ \mu g/mL$$

Therefore

$$C_{p\,max}^{ss} = \frac{13.5 \times 0.35}{0.35 - 0.12} \times \left\{\frac{e^{-0.12 \times 3.4}}{1 - e^{-0.12 \times 12}} - \frac{e^{-0.35 \times 3.4}}{1 - e^{-0.35 \times 12}}\right\}$$

$$C_{p\,max}^{ss} = 11.7 \ \mu g/mL$$

Predicted minimum concentration:

$$C_{p\,min}^{ss} = \frac{C_p^0 k_a}{k_a - k} \times \left\{\frac{e^{-0.12 \times 12}}{1 - e^{-0.12 \times 12}} - \frac{e^{-0.35 \times 12}}{1 - e^{-0.35 \times 12}}\right\}$$

$$C_{p\,min}^{ss} = 6.3 \ \mu g/mL$$

$\rightarrow$

CASE STUDY 12.2 (continued)

A dose of 675 mg b.d. was therefore recommended, which would give a predicted peak plasma concentration of 11.7 μg/mL and a predicted trough concentration of 6.3 μg/mL.

The infusion was continued overnight and stopped the following morning when oral dosing was commenced. After 3 days on the above dose, another level was taken at 11 h post dose, which was reported as 12.7 μg/mL. This was a trough concentration and it was twice the expected level of 6.3 μg/mL. This was probably due to the fact that Mr C.K.'s clearance had decreased and it was now actually approaching the initial population value for a nonsmoker.

From the IV data, Mr C.K.'s clearance was unusually high. The patient was not receiving any other drugs that influence theophylline clearance, he was a nonsmoker and the IV infusion was continuous. The apparent high initial clearance of theophylline cannot be explained.

This case illustrates the use of TDM in and during an acute exacerbation of asthma. The importance of measuring patient serum levels during oral mainten-ance therapy to reassess patient parameters is stressed since assessment of parameters during IV therapy (acute attack) may be misleading.

Note: Where a difference exists between theophylline clearance during IV therapy, following an acute exacerbation of asthma, and the clearance during oral therapy, following stabilisation, the latter clearance is often greater than the former, i.e. clearance improves as the patient's clinical condition improves. For no apparent reason, the reverse situation occurred in this patient.

CASE STUDY 12.3 Gentamicin

Mr E.L., a 49-year-old ex-brewery worker, was admitted to hospital generally feeling unwell and disoriented. His previous medical history showed that he had been a chronic alcohol user for previous two years and that he had a gas-trointestinal bleed 3 months previously. On examination, his height was 170 cm (5 ft 7 in.), his weight 72 kg; jaundice + + and no ascites. The diagnosis was that he was a chronic alcoholic, with possible hepatic encephalopathy and sepsis.

Biochemistry:

Serum urea	7 mmol/L (2.5–7.5 mmol/L)
Serum creatinine	86 μmol/L (50–130 μmol/L)
Albumin	35 g/L (30–46 g/L)

→

◗ CASE STUDY 12.3 (continued)

Total bilirubin	*121 μmol/L (>17 μmol/L)*
Serum sodium	*119 mmol/L (135–145 mmol/L)*

The plan is to start: Gentamicin IV 100 mg t.d.s.
　　　　　　　　　　　 Flucloxacillin IV 500 mg t.d.s.

Is this an appropriate dose of gentamicin?

Using a one compartment model:

　Ideal body weight = 66.1 kg

Estimated creatinine clearance using the Cockcroft and Gault (1976) equation:

　$CL_{cr} = 86$ mL/min

Estimated gentamicin clearance (Hardman *et al.*, 2001):

$$CL_{Gent} = (0.0438 \times 86) + (0.0036 \times 66.1) = 4 \text{ L/h}$$

Estimated $V_d^{ss} = 16.5$ L

It is important to note this patient does not have ascites. The volume of distribution of gentamicin is markedly increased in patients with ascites (Gill and Kern, 1979).

　Estimated $k = 0.2424 \text{ h}^{-1}$

Optimal interval (τ) for desired $C_{p\,max}^{ss} = 7$ mg/L and $C_{p\,min}^{ss} = 1$ mg/L. Using

$$\tau = \frac{\ln(C_{p\,max}^{ss}/C_{p\,min}^{ss})}{k}$$

$\tau = 8$ h

Hence 100 mg 8-hourly would achieve:

　Estimated $C_{p\,max}^{ss} = 7.1$ mg/L with $C_{p\,max}$ at 1 h = 5.6 mg/L
　Estimated $C_{p\,min}^{ss} = 1$ mg/L

Blood levels were taken on the fourth and fifth days of gentamicin treatment. Using enzyme immunoassay, results were:

	Serum creatinine	Total bilirubin	Gentamicin levels
Day 4	89 μmol/L	82 μmol/L	$C_{p\,max} = 8.9$ mg/L, sample time not specified
			$C_{p\,min} = 1.2$ mg/L
Day 5	93 μmol/L	77 μmol/L	$C_{p\,max} = 7.9$ mg/L, sample time not specified
			$C_{p\,min} = 1.8$ mg/L

→

How do the reported gentamicin levels compare to the estimated ones?
1. The reported levels for $C_{p\,max}$ are difficult to interpret because the sample time was not specified. However, assuming them to be correct, the patient's calculated $V\frac{d}{ss}$ would range from 12.9 L to 16.4 L, which agrees with initial estimates. Calculated drug clearance ranges from 3.2 to 3.5 L/h. This agrees closely with initial estimates.
2. The gentamicin injections were not given exactly 8-hourly, but at 0700 h, 1300 h and 2200 h, i.e. at intervals of 6, 9 and 9 h. The samples were supposedly taken on the 0700 h dose, which may also account for the discrepancy in the trough results compared with the estimated result. This particular problem has been highlighted by Scott *et al.* (1982).
3. The total bilirubin during these two days was 82 and 77 μmol/L. Wagner et al. (1983) reported two cases of interference of gentamicin levels leading to higher reported levels using the enzyme immunoassay, possibly owing to the bilirubin creating an opaque specimen. They recommend an alternative aminoglycoside assay method for patients with bilirubin concentrations greater than 68 μmol/L.

No more serum levels of gentamicin were taken because of the weekend and the patient was left on 100 mg t.d.s. On Friday (day 8 of gentamicin therapy), a serum creatinine was reported to be 162 μmol/L, but no action was taken. On Monday (day 11 of gentamicin therapy), a sample was taken for gentamicin and reported as follows at 0700 h:

$C_{p\,max}$	>17.6 mg/L
$C_{p\,min}$	>17.6 mg/L
Serum creatinine	563 μmol/L
Total bilirubin	49 mmol/L

What was the cause of E.L.'s decline in renal function?
A number of risk factors are associated with aminoglycoside nephrotoxicity (Evans *et al.*, 1986). Mr E.L. exhibited the following:

Patient factors:
*   *Sodium volume depletion.* The patient had a serum sodium ranging from 118 to 129 mmol/L during his therapy, so sodium depletion may have contributed to the nephrotoxicity of gentamicin. There is some evidence for a pure sodium deficiency increasing the risk of nephrotoxicity. However, volume depletion may also be a risk factor.

$\rightarrow$

CASE STUDY 12.3 (continued)

Drug factors:

- *Prior aminoglycoside exposure.* It was reported that E.L. had received a course of gentamicin during a previous admission to hospital. There is no convincing evidence that prior exposure causes subsequent toxicity.
- *Serum levels.* The raised trough on day 5 of treatment may have been responsible for the decline in renal function, or the decline in renal function may have already occurred, causing the trough to rise (the serum creatinine had already started to rise on day 5, suggesting that damage to renal function had occurred 2–9 days earlier). Care must be taken in interpreting the serum creatinine during E.L.'s admission in the early stages, as high bilirubin levels (greater than 27 μmol/L) may interfere with the assay for creatinine, giving falsely raised levels (Osberg and Hammond, 1978).
- *Other drugs.* Throughout this time period E.L. was receiving neomycin 1 g q.d.s. orally. A number of reports have suggested that oral neomycin may be absorbed in patients with liver disease (Kunin *et al.*, 1960; Last and Sherlock, 1960; Breen *et al.*, 1972).

Sadly no neomycin levels were performed and the patient was considered to have nephrotoxicity due to gentamicin. He went for a three-day course of dialysis to remove the gentamicin. The infection was treated eventually with a cephalosporin and the patient walked home with normal renal function two weeks later.

It is quite easy to attribute the decline in renal function to gentamicin, but it is very important not to forget the role of concurrent drug treatment.

CASE STUDY 12.4   Phenytoin

A 73-year-old man weighing 50 kg was admitted with a 2-week history of postherpetic neuralgia resistant to conventional analgesia. A trial of phenytoin and amitriptyline was considered appropriate.

What would be the expected phenytoin dose requirements for this patient?
The initial approach must rely on average population values for the Michaelis–Menten parameters V_m and K_m (Grasela *et al.*, 1983).

$\rightarrow$

◗ **CASE STUDY 12.4** (continued)

$K_m = 5.7$ mg/L
$V_m = [450 \,(\text{Weight}/70)^{0.6}]$ phenytoin sodium
$\quad = 450(50/70)^{0.6}$
$\quad = 368$ mg/day phenytoin sodium

(70 = average body weight in kg.)
N.B. When daily dose and V_m are expressed in the Michaelis–Menten equation, no correction for salt form is required provided both are expressed in the same terms.

$$\text{Daily dose} = \frac{V_m \times C_p^{ss}}{K_m + C_p^{ss}}$$

A therapeutic range for phenytoin in postherpetic neuralgia has not been established, but a range of 20–80 µmol/L has been suggested (Hatagandi *et al.*, 1976).
Take the initial target concentration as 40 µmol/L ≡ 10 mg/L.

$$\text{Daily dose} = \frac{368 \times 10}{5.7 + 10}$$
$$= 234 \text{ mg/day phenytoin sodium}$$

The expected dose requirements for this patient are likely to be 200–250 mg daily.
   Phenytoin was initially commenced at a dose of 200 mg daily. Analgesia remained poor and the dose was adjusted according to clinical response over the next two weeks to a final dose of 400 mg daily. Three days later, dizziness and ataxia developed.
   The patient's general condition had gradually deteriorated over this period owing, in part, to minimum protein and calorie intake. Investigations at this time revealed:

Albumin   23 g/L (35–50 g/L)
Serum phenytoin   58 µmol/L (20–80 µmol/L)

What is the likely cause of the observed dizziness and ataxia?
Dizziness, nystagmus, ataxia are predictable dose-related adverse effects of phenytoin. Nystagmus is generally the earliest symptom detected, and may occur between 60 and 120 µmol/L. Ataxia is usually seen above 120 µmol/L and alterations of consciousness may occur as levels exceed 160 µmol/L (Finn and Olanow, 1981).

→

CASE STUDY 12.4 (continued)

Why was toxicity observed in this patient at the apparently 'therapeutic level' of 58 μmol/L?

In hypoalbuminaemia, phenytoin binding is reduced and the total serum concentration may be misleading. Two approaches to this problem can be used.

1.   Direct assessment of the free phenytoin level. This can be performed using a simple ultrafiltration device that is commercially available. This approach may be useful in individual patients with a suspected binding abnormality (Baird-Lambert *et al.*, 1987).

   It is assumed that the effective range of free phenytoin is 2–8 μmol/L (i.e. the normal free component of the total therapeutic range).

   Measured free level = 10.4 μmol/L

2.   When free levels are not available, the following equation can be used to adjust the measured total phenytoin (Tozer and Winter, 1992).

$$\text{Adjusted phenytoin concentration} = \frac{\text{Observed total phenytoin concentration}}{0.9 \times \left(\dfrac{\text{Measured albumin}}{\text{Normal albumin (44 g/L)}} \right) + 0.1}$$

This equation assumes that the free fraction is 0.1 when the albumin is normal.

$$\text{Adjusted phenytoin concentration} = \frac{58}{0.9 \times (23/44) + 0.1}$$
$$= 102 \ \mu\text{mol/L}$$

The adjusted concentration can then be directly compared with the normal therapeutic range.

   Future dose adjustments may then be performed on the basis of the measured free level or the adjusted total level.

   Subsequent follow-up revealed that 250 mg daily maintained adequate analgesia without side-effects. The measured total concentration at this time was 26 μmol/L, which corresponded to an adjusted concentration of 46 μmol/L.

 CASE REPORT 12.5   Phenytoin

Mrs R.M., age 21 years, first presented on 15/07/1999 in the accident and emergency centre with viral encephalitis. She was discharged on phenytoin

→

> **CASE STUDY 12.5** (continued)

100 mg t.d.s. She weighed 60 kg. Following her discharge she had two fits in November. Two phenytoin measurements were made, which were 9.0 and 9.3 mg/L respectively.

Could a higher dose be given?
Calculate population V_m:

$$V_m = 450 \times (60/70)^{0.6} = 430 \text{ mg/day}$$

Calculate patient's V_m (using a K_m of 4 mg/L):

$$300 \text{ mg} = \frac{V_m \times 9 \text{ mg/L}}{4 \text{ mg/L} + 9 \text{ mg/L}}$$
$$V_m = 433 \text{ mg/day}$$

The two values are close, so the patient's V_m is used. Using this V_m, the level was calculated that would be produced by a dose of 350 mg. Thus:

$$350 \text{ mg} = \frac{V_m \times C_p^{ss}}{K_m + C_p^{ss}}$$
$$C_p^{ss} = 17 \text{ mg/L}$$

It was recommended that a dose of 350 mg could be administered. A level of 18.0 mg/L was recorded when a request for analysis (22/06/00) was later made. The patient still suffered from losses of consciousness, so at an outpatient appointment, 200 mg b.d. carbamazepine was added. A carbamazepine level was requested at the next visit (1/11/2000).
   Calculate carbamazepine level:

$$C_p^{ss} = \frac{D \times S \times F}{CL \times \tau}$$

Clearance was assumed to be 0.1 L/h/kg, so

$$C_p^{ss} = 2.7 \text{ mg/L}$$

This value was close to the assayed value of 2.5 mg/L. It was suggested to increase the dose to 600 mg/day, expected to produce a level of about 4 mg/L, possibly a little low. Over the next year, the neurologists decided, because of side-effects of hirsuteness and coarse features (not made known on the request

$\longrightarrow$

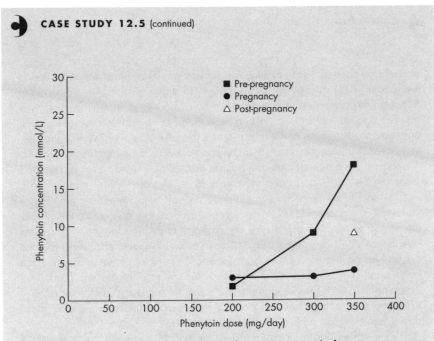

Figure 12.1 Phenytoin concentration for Mrs R.M. before pregnancy, during pregnancy and afterwards when phenytoin is given together with 60 mg phenobarbital.

forms), to *decrease* the dose of phenytoin to 200 mg/day, calculated to produce a level of 3.4 mg/L. In fact, an assay result of 2 mg/L was recorded. In spite of the low level of assayed phenytoin and predicted carbamazepine, the doses of drugs were not adjusted. Blood levels were again requested at a later date (09/01/02) and the results were still low at 2 mg/L and 4.25 mg/L for phenytoin and carbamazepine, respectively, and a repeated suggestion of a dose increase was not carried out because of the side-effect problem.

The patient was not seen again until September 2003, when it was reported that she was 4 weeks pregnant. She was still maintained on carbamazepine 600 mg/day and phenytoin 200 mg/day, relatively fit-free. Phenytoin level was checked on 23/10/03. It was 3 mg/L, and carbamazepine was 7 mg/L, still close to the predicted levels. She had three ictal episodes in the following few months, so her phenytoin was increased to 300 mg/day, but the level did not increase (see Figure 12.1). Carbamazepine was left unchanged. Non-compliance was ruled out, since drug levels are known to decrease during pregnancy (Chen *et al.*, 1982). The dose of phenytoin was thus increased to 350 mg and the level increased marginally to 4 mg/L.

Six months into the pregnancy, she developed an erythematous rash on the hands and feet and was advised to stop carbamazepine. Phenobarbital was

→

CASE STUDY 12.5 (continued)

started at a dose of 30 mg nightly. The patient was fit-free and was admitted to the labour ward on 16/06/04; a baby girl was delivered on 18/06/04. Although the phenobarbital levels were low (5.5 mg/L), breast feeding was advised against, since phenobarbital is reported to be excreted into breast milk and may produce high and variable levels (Kaneko *et al.*, 1979). Meanwhile, the patient's phenytoin level 6 days postpartum had increased to 6 mg/L. Although this is a modest increase, a more dramatic increase has been reported following the transition from partum to postpartum state (Freed *et al.*, 1986).

On 16/11/04 she was seen in the outpatients department complaining of tiredness. The phenytoin level was 9 mg/L, on 350 mg/day, while the phenobarbital level was 5.5 mg/L, now on 60 mg at night. The low phenytoin level (see Figure 12.1) compared with that of 4 years previously, probably reflected the interaction between phenobarbital and phenytoin. However, there have been conflicting reports on the importance of this interaction (Park and Breckenridge, 1981). The patient was seen in February 2005 with blood levels similar to before, but reasonably fit-free. It was decided to maintain these doses, avoiding the possible side-effects that may occur at higher levels.

It is not often that a patient can be followed for a considerable length of time, and one cannot be sure whether we have achieved the best for this patient. However, it does illustrate that although drug levels can be predicted fairly accurately by simple formulae, the additional information (often only known to the prescribing doctor) that is required before the final dose is arrived at may not be entirely evident to the kineticist, especially in the outpatient situation. It is essential to obtain as much clinical information as possible before giving a final definitive report.

On a more practical note, the problems of pregnancy and lactation while on antiepileptics (Nau *et al.*, 1982), and of a probable drug interaction are illustrated. Side-effect problems are highlighted, and this case emphasises that target ranges are only a guide to therapy. Remember that it is the patient who is being treated, not the drug levels.

CASE STUDY 12.6   Digoxin

Mrs A.S., a 78-year-old woman of height 160 cm (5 ft 3 in.), weighing 48 kg, was admitted to hospital at 0800 h on 2 May, after being found collapsed by

→

● **CASE STUDY 12.6** (continued)

neighbours that morning. The presenting complaints were that she had been unwell for a few weeks, and short of breath for the previous 6 months: PND 2/3 times per night; two pillows; she also has chest pain and ankle swelling.

Her GP two weeks before found abnormal pulse and prescribed digoxin 0.25 mg o.d. No loading dose was given; therapy started on Friday and she saw the GP the following Tuesday. As there were no problems it was decided to continue on that dose.

There was a 3-day history of nausea, no vomiting and past medical history of arthritic knee.

Drugs on admission:	Digoxin	250 µg o.d.
	Diclofenac	50 mg b.d. for right knee
CVS:	Pulse	45 beats/min
	BP	130/80 mmHg
	JVP	↓
ECG:		Sinus bradycardia S-T segment depression in V_4
Biochemistry:	Serum sodium	135 mmol/L
	Serum potassium	5.2 mmol/L
	Serum urea	16.3 mmol/L
	Serum creatinine	108 µmol/L
Digoxin level at 1600 h, 2 May:	4.27 ng/mL	
Diagnosis: digoxin toxicity		

The question asked by the medical team was whether this lady should have been given that dose of digoxin

Using population data (Kelman et al., 1982):

$$CL_{Dig} \text{ (L/h)} = [0.06 CL_{cr} \text{ (mL/min)}] + (0.02 \times weight)$$

From the Cockcroft and Gault (1976) equation:

$$CL_{cr} = 28.65 \text{ mL/min}$$

Weight = 48 kg. Hence

$$CL_{Dig} = 2.68 \text{ L/h}$$

Giving 250 µg daily, predicted average plasma level (C_p^{ss}) is

$$C_p^{ss} = \frac{250 \times 0.63}{24 \times 2.68} = 2.5 \text{ µg/L compared to 4.27 µg/L reported.}$$

→

● **CASE STUDY 12.6** (continued)

Assuming the reported level is correct:

$$CL_{Dig} = \frac{250 \times 0.63}{24 \times 4.27} = 1.54\,L/h$$

compared to 2.68 L/h (population).

Reasons for reduced the clearance include:

- *Deteriorating renal function.* This was possible as this lady was given diclofenac, which could have caused a decrease in renal blood flow and/or glomerular filtration (Clive and Stoff, 1984).
- *Other drugs being co-administered that reduce clearance.* There was no evidence of any other drugs being taken.
- *Increase in the bioavailability.* If the bioavailability had increased from the assumed 0.63 to a maximum of 1.0, this still would not account for the observed high plasma level.
- *Altered thyroid function.* There was no clinical evidence of hypothyroidism that would cause a decrease in clearance and volume of distribution. This was later confirmed chemically.
- *The sample may not have been taken at the correct time.* Sample time was greater than 6 h and this can be ruled out as a problem.
- *Noncompliance.* Compliance with the regimen could be a problem and she may have taken two digoxin tablets instead of digoxin plus diclofenac that morning.

At this stage, in view of the present situation, all drugs were stopped and it was suggested that a further level be done. A level 6 days later was reported as:

Digoxin   0.49 ng/mL
Serum creatinine   89 μmol/L

Since she had had no digoxin for 6 days, it is possible to calculate the elimination rate constant k_e:

$$k = \frac{\ln(4.27/0.49)}{144} = 0.01503\,h^{-1}$$

Estimate V_d as

$$V_d = (3.12 \times CL_{cr}) + (3.84 \times weight)$$

CL_{cr} has not significantly changed, but using the more recent serum creatinine of 89 μmol/L:

$$CL_{cr} = 34.8\,mL/min$$

compared to the previous value of 28.7 mL/min. Therefore,

→

> ● **CASE STUDY 12.6** (continued)
>
> $$V_d = (3.12 \times 34.8) + (3.84 \times 48) = 292.9\,L$$
>
> Hence,
>
> $$\text{Patient clearance of digoxin} = 0.01503 \times 292.9 = 4.4\,L/h$$
>
> If this is assumed to be the clearance of digoxin on starting therapy:
>
> $$\text{Predicted } C_p^{ss} = \frac{250 \times 0.63}{24 \times 4.4} = 1.5\,ng/mL$$
>
> which would have been more appropriate for this patient.
> Mrs A.S. was discharged from hospital a week later taking paracetamol only.
>
> **Practice points**
> 1. The GP had not given a loading dose of digoxin and asked to see her after only 5 days – at this stage the patient was not at steady state, and he should have waited at least 10 days before reviewing her.
> 2. The diclofenac may have had some small effect on renal function, but not of clinical importance in this case (however, it should never be overlooked).
> 3. Compliance must be very suspect in this case and must therefore influence future management.

References

Case study 12.1

Kelman A W, Whiting B, Bryson S M (1982). OPT: a package of computer programs for parameter optimisation in clinical pharmacokinetics. *Br J Clin Pharmacol* 14(2): 247–256.

Case study 12.3

Breen K J, Bryant R E, Levinson J D, Schenker S (1972). Neomycin absorption in man. *Ann Int Med* 76: 211–218.

Cockcroft D W, Gault M H (1976). Prediction of creatinine clearance from serum creatinine. *Nephron* 16: 31–41.

Evans W E, Schentag J J, Jusko W J, eds. (1986). *Applied Pharmacokinetics: Principles of Therapeutic Drug Monitoring*, 2nd edn. Spokane: Applied Therapeutics.

Gill M A, Kern I N (1979). Altered gentamicin distribution in ascitic patients. *Am J Hosp Pharm* 36: 1704–1706.

Hardman J G, Limbird L E, Goodman L S, Gilman A, eds. *Goodman and Gilman's The Pharmacological Basis of Therapeutics*, 10th edn. New York: McGraw-Hill.

Kunin C M, Chalmers M D, *et al.* (1960). Absorption of orally administered neomycin and kanamycin. *N Engl J Med* 262(8): 380–385.

Last P M, Sherlock S (1960). Systematic absorption of orally administered neomycin in liver disease. *N Engl J Med* 262(8): 385–389.

Osberg I M, Hammond K B (1978). A solution to the problem of bilirubin interference with kinetic Jaffe method for serum creatinine. *Clin Chem* 24: 1169–1170.

Scott D K, Davey P G, Gonda I, Harpur E S (1982). Aminoglycoside trough levels: a source of error. *Lancet* (21 Aug): 441–442.

Wagner J C, Misinski J, Slama T G (1983). Falsely elevated aminoglycoside serum levels in jaundiced patients. *Drug Intell Clin Pharm* 17: 544–546.

Case study 12.4

Baird-Lambert J, Manglick M P, Wall M, Buchanan N (1987). Identifying patients who might benefit from free phenytoin monitoring. *Ther Drug Monit* 9: 134–138.

Finn A L, Olanow M D (1981). Phenytoin: Therapeutic use and serum concentration monitoring. In: Taylor W J, Finn A L, eds. *Individualizing Drug Therapy – Practical Applications of Drug Monitoring*. New York: Gross, Townsend, Frank, 64–85.

Grasela T H, Sheiner L B, Rambeck B, *et al.* (1983). Steady state pharmacokinetics of phenytoin from routinely collected patient data. *Clin Pharmacokinet* 8: 355–364.

Hatagandi V S, Boas R A, Richards E G (1976). Post-herpetic neuralgia: management with anti-epileptic and tricyclic drugs. In: Bonica J J, Albe-Fessard D G, eds. *Proceedings of the First World Congress on Pain. Advances in Pain Research and Therapy*, vol. 1. New York: Raven Press, 583–587.

Tozer T N, Winter M E (1992). Phenytoin: In: Evans W E, Schentag J J, Jusko W J, eds. *Applied Pharmacokinetics: Principles of Therapeutic Drug Monitoring*, 3rd edn. Vancouver: Applied Therapeutics.

Case study 12.5

Chen S-S, Perucca E, Lee J-N, Richens A (1982). Serum protein binding and free concentration of phenytoin and phenobarbitone in pregnancy. *Br J Clin Pharmacol* 13: 547–552.

Freed C R, Gal J, Manchestser D K (1985). Dosage of phenytoin during pregnancy. *JAMA* 253: 2833–2844.

Kaneko S, Sato T, Suzuki K (1979). The levels of anticonvulsants in breast milk. *Br J Clin Pharmacol* 7: 624–626.

Nau H, Kuhnz W, Egger H-J, Rating D, Helge H (1982). Anticonvulsants during pregnancy and lactation. Transplacental, maternal and neonatal pharmacokinetics. *Clin Pharmacokinet* 7: 508–543.

Park B K, Breckenridge A M (1981). Clinical implications of enzyme induction and enzyme inhibition. *Clin Pharmacokinet* 6: 1–24.

Case study 12.6

Clive D M, Stoff J S (1984). Renal syndromes associated with nonsteroidal anti-inflammatory drugs. *N Engl J Med* 310: 583.

Cockcroft D W, Gault M H (1976). Prediction of creatinine clearance from serum creatinine. *Nephron* 16: 31–41.

Kelman A W, Whiting B, Bryson S M (1982). OPT: a package of computer programs for parameter optimisation in clinical pharmacokinetics. *Br J Clin Pharmacol* 14(2): 247–256.

Index

renal impairment (*cont'd*)
elderly patients, 62–3
lithium clearance, 186–7
lithium therapy-related, 171
phamacokinetic alterations, 57
absorption, 58
bioavailability, 58
distribution, 58–9
excretion, 61
metabolism, 59–61
phenytoin, 198, 200
therapeutic drug monitoring, 53–4, 63
renal replacement therapy, 63–8, 74
case study, 75–6
drug removal, 64–6, 66
dialyser characteristics, 65
drug characteristics, 65
loading doses, 66–7
maintenance dose administration, 67–8
phamacokinetic models, 64
postdialysis redistribution phenomena, 65
postdialysis replacement dose, 64
renal transplantation, 77, 217, 218, 221, 222, 224
rifampicin, 97

salicylates, 4, 103
salivary drug concentrations, 51
lithium monitoring, 172
salt factor
digoxin, 137
intravenous infusions, 18, 21
orally administred drugs, 23
steady state conditions, 17
theophylline, 152, 152
schizophrenia, 169
seizures, 193–4, 197
classification, 194
definition, 194
selective serotonin-reuptake inhibitors (SSRIs), lithium interactions, 185
sieving coefficient, 67–8
simple partial seizures, 194
single intravenous bolus injection, 12–13, 37
single oral dose, 21–2, 22, 37
smoking, theophylline phamacokinetics, 154, 157

sodium valproate, 194, 205–6
adverse effects, 206
drug interactions, 50, 202, 206, 209
mode of action, 206
plasma protein binding, 50
use in pregnancy, 206
software, 51
spironolactone, digoxin interaction, 143
status epilepticus, 195, 200, 207, 210
steady state conditions, 82
administration/elimination relationship, 17–18
average plasma concentration, 17, 38
determinants of time to reach steady state, 14
dose effects, 13, 14
dosing interval effects, 14, 15
half-life relationship, 18, 18
intravenous infusions, 18–21, 19
decay following discontinuation, 19–20, 20
following loading dose, 20–1, 21
maximum plasma concentration, 17
minimum plasma concentration, 17
multiple intravenous dosing, 13, 13
levels at times within dosing interval, 16–17, 16
levels following commencement of dosing, 14–16, 15
nonlinear phamacokinetics, 32–4, 32, 33, 35
plasma protein binding influence, 36, 41
orally administred drugs
average plasma concentration, 26
maximum plasma concentration, 25
minimum plasma concentration, 25
plasma levels prior to steady state, 23–4, 24
sulphonylureas, 103
suxamethonium, 104

target range *see* therapeutic range
teratogenesis
carbamazepine, 203
lithium, 179
sodium valproate, 206
tetracyclines, lithium interactions, 180